STUDIES IN HISTORY, ECONOMICS AND PUBLIC LAW

EDITED BY THE FACULTY OF POLITICAL SCIENCE
OF COLUMBIA UNIVERSITY

Number 287

SOCIAL FACTORS IN MEDICAL PROGRESS

TABLE OF CONTENTS

	PAGE
INTRODUCTION	7

PART I
FACTORS WHICH RETARD THE DIFFUSION OF MEDICAL DISCOVERIES

CHAPTER I
Factors which Retard the Diffusion of Innovations 11

CHAPTER II
Conservatism in Medicine, a Perspective 20

CHAPTER III
Opposition to Dissection 34

CHAPTER IV
Opposition to Harvey's Theory of the Circulation of the Blood .. 44

CHAPTER V
Reception of Auenbrugger's Theory of Percussion 51

CHAPTER VI
Opposition to Vaccination 53

CHAPTER VII
Opposition to Holmes and Semmelweis 66

CHAPTER VIII
Opposition to Pasteur and His Discoveries 71

CHAPTER IX
Opposition to the Doctrine of Antisepsis 80

CONTENTS

CHAPTER X
Opposition to Asepsis 90

CHAPTER XI
Summary 93

PART II

THE NATURE OF MEDICAL PROGRESS

CHAPTER I
Biography in Medical History 97

CHAPTER II
The Dependence of a Discovery upon the Existing Knowledge . . 100

CHAPTER III
Multiple Inventions and Discoveries in the History of Medicine . . 108

BIBLIOGRAPHY 128

INDEX 135

INTRODUCTION

SOCIOLOGISTS have recently been investigating the nature of the behavior of culture during the process of change. Many questions have presented themselves for study. To what extent and why are innovations or changes in culture resisted? What are the psychological and sociological factors involved in this resistance? What is the nature of cultural growth? Are gifted individuals responsible for progress? Would progressive change have come about without the work of the particular individuals now accredited with the inventions and discoveries? An attempt has been made here to answer these and other related questions by an analysis of some of the phases of the history of medicine. This field was chosen for such an inquiry because in measuring the value of an innovation, the subjective factor can be eliminated to a greater degree than when dealing with the subject matter of politics, religion, art or economics.

The present inquiry is concerned with two aspects of cultural change as it occurs in the field of medicine, the first, an analysis of the psychological and sociological factors which retard the diffusion of innovations, and the second, the nature of progress in medicine. These questions will be treated separately in Part I and Part II respectively.

Hypotheses suggested by previous sociologists as to why change is resisted, were submitted to the test of evidence derived from an analysis of the controversies over innovations in the history of medicine. The result was a revised and supplemented list of factors involved in retarding change which is presented in the first chapter. Preliminary to a detailed critically historical analysis of the reasons for opposition to specific important discoveries, the distinctive characteristics of the problem of conservatism in medicine are described as a setting for the later discussion. Controversies over dissection, the theory of the circulation of the blood, percussion, vaccination, the theory of puerperal fever as a contagious disease, Pasteur's discoveries, antisepsis and asepsis are then examined with the purpose of discerning the retarding factors involved in each instance, and the degree of intensity of these factors. The brief concluding summary enumerates the factors present in the specific controversies analyzed.

Part II is concerned with the problem of cultural accumulation in the history of medicine or the nature of the growth of medical knowledge. The treatment deals with inquiries regarding the extent to which an individual contributes to any invention or discovery in medicine and the degree of the dependence of discoveries upon prior knowledge in the field of medicine and upon developments in fields independent of medicine. This resolves itself into a discussion of the problem of whether inventions or discoveries in medicine would have been made irrespective of the individuals who are now heralded as the innovators. The significance of the many multiple discoveries in the history of medicine will be analysed in this connection and a list of such discoveries appended.

The term culture will be used throughout the book as it is defined by anthropologists and sociologists as the equivalent of social heritage or accumulated knowledge.

PART I
FACTORS WHICH RETARD THE DIFFUSION OF MEDICAL DISCOVERIES

CHAPTER I

FACTORS WHICH RETARD THE DIFFUSION OF INNOVATIONS

CONTROVERSIES which have followed the introduction of medical discoveries have been analyzed in this inquiry in the light of previous sociological studies which have set forth hypotheses about the character of the psychological and sociological factors which resist change.[1] These hypotheses, revised and supplemented after a review of the evidence derived from the history of medicine, are presented here to orientate the reader in the method of approach of this study. The illustrative data from the history of medicine from which these hypotheses were formulated will subsequently be given.

Among the chief factors which seem to determine the rate of social change, by influencing the incorporation or rejection of an innovation, is vested interest. In the following discussion, this concept will be used both in the restricted sense of economic interests which resist changes that would affect adversely the advantage obtaining under the conditions held prior to the innovation, and also in reference to that less tangible vested interest bound up with the struggle to retain status, reputation and prestige. The economic interests are possessed of vast effective power due to the control these interests have over the press and educational and political institutions and through the funds at their disposal to mould resistant attitudes through propaganda. The vested interest of personal self-fulfillment functions through the attachment of an " emotional tone " to the existing process which makes

[1] See especially: Wm. F. Ogburn, *Social Change*, 1923, pp. 145-196.

devotion to it and resistance to any substitute for it in the form of an innovation, unreasoning and unreceptive to any scientific proof of the latter's superior effectiveness. The older form is suffused with a value and meaning which it does not actually possess; loyalty is justified and the newer process or method is withstood.

The "power of tradition" is a general descriptive concept that is used to characterize a phase of hostility to change. It implies the social attitude that the customary ways of doing things are better in spite of all their failings because they have been tried, while there may be unknown dangers lurking in the new procedure. Conservatism seems to be concomitant with inability to cope with problems through lack of knowledge, whatever the cause of the ignorance may be. This does not imply that those equipped with knowledge will always respond favorably to innovations. There does not appear to be a positive correlation between knowledge and receptiveness, because the other factors such as vested interest and habit counteract that asset. But, on the other hand, ignorance creates apprehension which intensifies caution. The fear reaction in the presence of the unknown is especially evident in phases of human activity that involve control over human life and welfare, where disaster can easily be ascribed to the innovation because of lack of actual scientific proof. The desire for security, opposing change, cuts across and inhibits the desire of fresh stimulation that welcomes change. Furthermore, the traditional mode of acting has already been incorporated and adapted to other aspects of culture. An innovation implies a new orientation and adjustment, perhaps a far-reaching revision of many phases of the existing culture. This in turn may involve again the vested interests concerned with perpetuating *status quo,* which aid in intensifying the desire for security.

Another factor in opposition to change is the reverence

for authority prevalent among the majority of people who are neither equipped nor acquainted with the experimental or scientific method of verifying data. The lack of ability to analyze proof as a criterion of truth may perhaps be ascribed to faulty educational technique which has emphasized the perpetuation of tradition rather than methods of inquiry. The diversity and complexity of knowledge seem even to demand the acceptance of the principle of authority in the majority of judgments of those equipped with the technique of examining evidence. The question of use of authority involves the choice of authority and the competence of individuals to weigh the relative merits of conflicting authorities. In general, this seems to lead to the glorification of the individual who represents the traditional approach and is " safe ".

The educational system intensifies the " power of tradition ", reflecting the domination and interests of the class in power, not only because of the emphasis on content rather than method, mentioned above, but because of the inertia in changing the content to conform with the ever-changing accumulation in and revision of knowledge. The " mind set " of the teachers, fixed by the traditional knowledge prior to the innovation and intensified by the mechanical elements involved in the present educational system, which afford little opportunity to teachers to continue their research, are to some extent responsible. The economic cost of changing text books, of transforming laboratory technique to the new requirements, the expenditure and mechanical delays involved in expanding the faculty by adding specialists in the new field, often cause the educational institutions to lag far behind the accumulating knowledge. There seems to exist also, caution lest the institution be discredited by an innovation that may prove illusory, and a fear on the part of the administration that the publicity involved in attacking the traditional attitude and the vested interests concerned, will work hardship on the institution.

The psychological factor of habit strengthens the " power of tradition ". The types of behavior, conditioned in the traditional way, continue even after the innovation is accepted conceptually. The development of new habits involves an expenditure of effort and a temporary readjustment of the individual. This is avoided as long as the present mode of thinking and behavior is in any way effective. The reconditioning of concepts and of behavior, necessary for the acceptance of an innovation is difficult, requiring conscious direction and control. The easier alternate response by an individual with habits already formed, confronted with the necessity of adapting himself to an innovation, is to act in the habitual way and then to rationalize his action, that is, justify his conduct by excuses which sanction it.

Especially does the change seem to be resisted and rationalizations made if the innovation involves personal inconvenience in the form of temporary pain, or the necessity for more precision and accuracy. The avoidance of pain is a psychological factor which often enters into conflict with an innovation. The desire also to expend the least possible amount of energy in accomplishing a task, inclines many individuals to resist complicated and exacting innovations, and to continue the old methods which have certain utility, even if they are not as efficient as the new. All cultural survivals can be found to have some utility in the sense that they satisfy some human want, even though they may be superseded in effectiveness by some later process.

Initiators and proponents of inventions and discoveries deviate from the mode of collective behavior of the group, which in order to protect itself, uses forms of social pressure to exact conformity.[1] Collective activity is expedited through orderliness and definiteness, based on acceptance of the existing social pattern, and the established habit reactions

[1] F. H. Giddings, *Studies in the Theory of Human Society*, p. 197 *et seq.*

of the individuals composing the group. The "consciousness of kind" of the group results in resentment against changes which disturb the orderliness of the social organizations and imply even a temporary social confusion. Fundamental innovations implying as they do a revision of customary behavior and a revaluation of social habits, create maladjustments which upset the routine behavior patterns and disarrange the regularity of social activity. They are therefore resisted in order that *status quo,* which has the appearance of orderliness, may be preserved.

This social pressure may be effected by certain patent devices. The invention or discovery is often completely ignored by the group, which in order to avoid the unpleasant, refuses to recognize its existence by even discussing it. The innovator is always placed militantly on the defensive. Ridicule and sneers directed against the innovator, as well as the innovation, cow the timid. Derogatory personal remarks, innuendoes that the innovator is advertising himself from motives of egotism and vanity, insinuations that he is obsessed with one pet idea which causes him to exaggerate its importance, all aim to discount the discovery and force its advocates to conform. Another discrediting device is to emphasize and give publicity to minor errors in the discovery, neglecting entirely to mention the main purport of the innovation. Inasmuch as no innovation when first presented is entirely perfect, such caviling criticisms are effective in obscuring and discounting the importance of the discovery, delaying its acceptance and perpetuating the customary procedure. Furthermore, as no innovation is entirely new, and a discovery is very often made simultaneously by two or more men, the defenders of the intrenched system often attempt to detract from the value of the discovery by controversies over priority.

Many individuals are particularly sensitive to social approval and the tendency is to avoid such activity as will involve one in controversy and conflict with others. Since the individual who interferes with and disrupts the normal orderly functioning of custom, stimulates the resentment of the group and provokes the use of the devices of social pressure outlined above, many are discouraged from projecting or supporting innovations. Reputation, social and economic standing are involved, and conformity offers relief from the acrimonious altercations in which an innovator must engage. Social pressure, supplemented by the individual's desire to avoid the unpleasant, thus acts as a powerful resistant to change.

Even when vested interests and authority are not actively opposed to a change, and the innovation does not involve a decided revision of individual and group behavior, the established tends to persist. This phase of cultural inertia or slowness of social change may be ascribed to the purely mechanical problem of diffusing knowledge. Many people must adopt a procedure before it can be said to be accepted, and this requires time to effect. The discovery, made by a specialist, is published in one of many periodicals in the field, reaching a negligible number of readers. Of these only a few who are interested transmit the information to others, and so the discovery becomes known to an ever-widening circle of specialists. This diffusion, even among those especially concerned with the innovation is slow. The difficulty is intensified when the problem of reaching those not immediately interested is considered. The gaps between the specialists and others even in the same field, are becoming increasingly wide as knowledge accumulates and related subjects are becoming more and more differentiated. The technical terminology, developing rapidly in each specialty, is difficult for the non-specialist to comprehend, and the communication of the discovery to the larger group is thereby retarded even when the discovery is given wide publicity. The diffusion of knowledge of an innovation among those entirely uninformed constitutes an even greater task.

Money often plays an important role in retarding cultural change. The fear of economic loss may restrain the innovator from projecting, the publisher from printing, the educational institution from supporting and the prospective user from investing in the innovation. When the innovation necessitates the expenditure of money for new implements and equipment, the fact that many people lack the necessary capital often prevents its general reception.

When an innovation is made in any field of culture, it may be in immediate conflict with some other established or competing activity which purposes to accomplish the same end. If one conceives of culture as composed of interrelated units, certain units within each phase of culture appear to be struggling with one another for survival irrespective of the individuals supporting them. In the same manner an innovation in one phase of culture such as medicine, may conflict with a seemingly unrelated unit in culture, a church doctrine, a theological concept, a political ideal. Although these conflicts take place through and are dramatized by the medium of personalities, yet they are actually struggles between different ideas, techniques, modes of activity and institutions. The rate of diffusion of an innovation is affected by the extent to which it must compete with units in its own field and with units in other fields.

The struggle between an innovation and other units in culture, is often complicated by the personality and affiliations of the innovator. The individual is intimately identified by others with his discovery or invention and its diffusion is retarded if he arouses resentment by personality traits disagreeable to those who must be convinced of the efficacy of the innovation. Recognizing the fact that it is much more dramatic and therefore more effective to discredit a personality than to refute an idea, opponents of innovation often use personality attacks as expedients to hide the actual causes which motivate them.

The above factors involved in retarding change may be classified roughly as psychological, cultural, mechanical, and personality factors. The psychological factors discerned are: first, the tendency to suffuse an habitual mode of activity with an "emotional tone" to justify the continuance of the habit rather than adopt another type of behavior. This process may be characterized as the development of a psychological vested interest. Second, there is fear reaction in the presence of the unknown; third, the persistence of habit reactions due to the difficulty of reconditioning behavior patterns; fourth, the avoidance of pain and the unpleasant; fifth, the mechanism of rationalization; sixth, social pressure enforced by the "consciousness of kind" of the group. The cultural factors are: first, economic vested interests; second, the power of personal and established institutional authority; third, ignorance; fourth, the role of money; fifth, the conflict of one phase of culture with another within the same field of activity and with other fields. The mechanical factors are: first, the difficulties of diffusing knowledge due to the mass of individuals to be moved; second, the mechanical difficulties of effecting change in institutional activity. Personality factors are often brought into play through the development of personality conflicts during the controversy.

The factors listed can only be isolated from one another conceptually. Actually, they are intimately interrelated and overlapping as the previous discussion indicates and as the following data from the history of medicine will substantiate. For example, authority acquires its power from such psychological factors as habit, fear, and the avoidance of pain and from such cultural factors as economic vested interests and ignorance. Economic vested interest is interrelated with fear of loss of power and the avoidance of pain. When conflicts between phases of culture and between individuals occur all the other factors listed are likely to be brought into play. The psychological factors also are intimately bound up with one another. These factors may however, be distinguished and isolated to permit a clearer and more graphic interpretation of the behavior of culture during the process of change.

CHAPTER II

CONSERVATISM IN MEDICINE, A PERSPECTIVE

RESISTANCE to the introduction of innovations in medicine cannot be adequately interpreted without an understanding of the status of medicine as a science and the attending predicament of the medical man. It will be the purpose of this chapter, to give this requisite background for the later discussion of resistance to change in medicine, to classify briefly certain historical instances of conservatism and to characterize the part played by laymen in medical conservatism.

In medicine, dealing as it does with the human organism in relation to its complex environment, it is difficult to speak with certainty of " proof ". Nothing can be held to be absolutely verified and " true ", due to the multiplicity of factors involved. Edmond Hobhouse, after a careful analysis of the scientific basis of medicine, stated that the intrinsic difficulties of medicine

can never be entirely removable, because even if we regard a complete knowledge of what we have called the unknown physiological constants, (i. e. of the operative processes of the ultimate tissue elements and their causation) as finally attainable, those processes are conditioned by the inherited (variable) tendencies of the organism of which they are specifically the vital energising basis, and these latter we have endeavored to show, are on the most hopeful theory incalculable, so that in the last resort, whatever be the balance of probabilities in our favor (i. e. the individual will conform within certain widish limits to a definite physiological type) the results of medicine in any given case must rest on an empirical determination with respect to the individual and therefore be to some degree uncertain.[1]

Dyce Duckworth expressed a similar view in the number of the *British Medical Journal* devoted to an analysis of " quackery ":

In so far as modern medicine is scientific, it stands by itself with problems before it which no other science has to face and unravel. We have often to act, sometimes promptly, on probabilities, with no scientific indications to guide us. The personal factor in the individual, not always easy to recognize, has to be reckoned with, and each patient is a new and special problem for us at the bedside.[2]

Even apart from the problem of individual variation, the exact scientific data of medicine are meagre compared to the factors which are still empirically determined.

When one surveys the field of medicine and observes the chaos of conflicting opinions as to the etiology and treatment of diseases, he recognizes the plight of the physician who is desirous of being progressive. In the field of drug therapy, the physician is especially perplexed. New drug and serum products are put on the market, enticingly advertised, endorsed by excellent authorities, substantiated ostensibly by experimental data. To investigate adequately the real value of these innovations is a prodigious task which is beyond the power of even the exceptional physician. His choice must be guided by faith in authority and by his experience with the drug after using it upon his patients. Meeting frequent disillusionment, he becomes cautious. If the remedy is suc-

[1] Edmond Hobhouse, *The Scientific Basis of Medicine*, Oxford, 1895, p. 52.
[2] Dyce Duckworth, " Rational Empiricism and Scientific Medicine," *British Medical Journal*, May 27, 1911, p. 1218. See also Paul De Kruif, *Our Medicine Men*, 1922, *passim*.

cessful, he is never entirely sure that his reasoning is not *post hoc ergo propter hoc*, for he cannot determine whether the regenerative powers of the tissues of the body would not have restored health without the application of the drug. In addition to being forced to select the valuable from all the new preparations resulting from the rapid development of organic chemistry, he finds that contemporary destructive and critical pharmacodynamics is rejecting vast numbers of the alleged remedies upon which his predecessors pinned their faith. Constructive pharmacology is in its infancy and yet remedies may now " be enumerated in units where they were once counted in scores ".[1] The tendency of recent pharmacology toward simplification and specificity will, in the end, facilitate the work of the physician, but at present, with most of the old reliable drugs under suspicion, he is in a quandary. The rejection of the old drugs by the research worker leaves him perplexed. Put on the defensive, he becomes conservative, and often persists in using the old alleged remedies even after their efficacy has been disproven thoroughly, because of his " mind-set " and habit reaction.

In all fields, the very foundations of medical theory are being revolutionized. Conflicting theories are endorsed with equal vehemence by equally competent authorities. The following quotation indicates the controversial background in which the physician finds himself.

The trend of recent medicine from the bacterial theory of disease toward the biochemical is strongly marked in Ehrlich's work. The fallibility of the many tests for differentiating the pseudo-typhoid, pseudo-tubercle, and pseudo-diphtheritic bacilli, the fact that only a fixed laboratory strain of a given bacillus is definitely pathogenic, the uncertainty of the behavior of many

[1] F. H. Garrison, *History of Medicine*, 3rd ed., pp. 703-4. The French clinicians, Huchard and Fiessinger, have limited actual drug therapy to some twenty remedies or groups of remedies.

bacilli in fermenting sugar-media, the puzzling mutations and polymorphisms, such as Penfold's *Bacillus coli mutabile,* which generates incontinently typhoid or coli germs, the apparent changes of one bacillus into another, the effect of meteorological conditions on insulin fermentation, the strange vagaries of agglutination and of Wasserman tests, all show the inadequacy of our present knowledge and how little we really know of intracellular chemistry. As in applied sanitary science, opinion is divided between those who maintain that the prevention of disease and mortality rests mainly with the individual, and those who believe that causation and prevention are multiplex and largely external to the individual; so in the infantile science of epidemiology, just emerging from the descriptive stage, there are already two schools, one relying on the bacterial theory of infection for its data, and one, headed by Crookshank, harking back to the Sydenham doctrine of epidemic constitutions, family relationships between diseases and external (cosmic and telluric) phenomena as contributory causes of epidemics.[1]

The pediatrician was told by Biedert that casein was harmful, by A. Czerny that fats were harmful, by Escherich, that intestinal bacteria were harmful, by Rotch that proteids were harmful, and Finkelstein maintained that salt and sugar intoxication was the basis of infantile nutritive disorders, a theory which he later abandoned in part.[2] When the gynecologist studies the history of his field, he sees a series of " crazes " and always a tendency to follow prevailing fashion. The uterine displacement craze, when every gynecologist invented or modified a pessary for the treatment of backache or pelvic pain, was followed by a pelvic cellulitis craze which was widely taken up until it was exploded. Oöphorectomy, clitoridectomy, inflammation of the os and cervix uteri, excision of the uterus and its appendages, operations for extrauterine pregnancy and Cesarean section, all were once preva-

[1] Garrison, *ibid.,* p. 748.
[2] Garrison, *ibid.,* p. 674.

lent fashions.[1] Discarded surgical practices once legitimate are multitudinous.[2] Phlebotomy or bloodletting, once the dominant therapeutic procedure, is now entirely abandoned. " What is called quackery at the present day often represents what was orthodox medicine two or three centuries ago ".[3]

The medical man who is conscious of the fact that fads and fancies in medicine and surgery have followed each other in transitory popularity and who recognizes that the stupendous accumulation of medical knowledge has become too great for him to master, becomes conservative. The conservative tendency resulting from this inability to cope with the multitudinous discoveries and inventions in medicine, is clearly brought out by a quotation from Dyce Duckworth:

It cannot be disputed that it has been difficult, and sometimes impossible, for those fully engaged in practice to keep pace with the progress in medical knowledge in the last twenty-five years. Discoveries and new methods for diagnosis and treatment have been laid before us with increasing rapidity, some of the greatest value, others of little or none; and amongst the latter are the novelties which are almost daily pressed on our attention after the manner of a Parisian *modiste* with the gentler sex. To acquire any practical knowledge of these would make a heavy claim on the attention of those who ventured to adopt them, and the result would be almost inevitably to displace some well acquired and certified methods of practice and to upset principles which have been well established by long clinical experience.[4]

[1] Garrison, *ibid.*, pp. 650-651.
[2] See O. S. Steiner, *Ohio State Medical Journal*, vol. xvii, pp. 170-1 for a protracted list. See also, G. F. Butler, "Cubism in Medicine," *Illinois Medical Journal*, vol. xxxix, p. 250 (1921); F. B. Wynn, "Fads and Fashions of Medical Practice," *Journal of Indiana State Medical Association*, vol. xiv, p. 117 *et seq.*
[3] *British Medical Journal*, May 27, 1911, p. 1251.
[4] *British Medical Journal*, May 27, 1911, p. 1217.

The physician's conservatism is intensified by his desire to guard against the tremendous influence of mass suggestion, on the part of physicians and the general public. It is further heightened by his fear of losing his professional status by being classed as a " quack " or " faddist ", thus suffering economic loss.

His recourse is to authority, where the tendency is to encounter even greater conservatism. The history of medicine is replete with instances where the most prominent authorities of the time, through their influence, retarded innovations. Riolan, Caspar Hoffman and other authorities of Harvey's day opposed the theory of the circulation of the blood.[1] Van Swieten, De Haen, Sprengel, Vogel, Baldinger, contemporary authorities of Auenbrugger ignored his book the *Percussion of the Chest* which was not appreciated until the time of Corvisart.[2] When McDowell published his work on ovariotomy in 1817, all authorities who knew of it condemned it. Diderot was thrown into the Bastille for three months for showing how the blind survive in the struggle for life by the supreme adaptability of their four remaining senses, and suggesting the possibility of teaching them to read and write by the sense of touch.[3] The French Academy ridiculed Desmoulins' discovery of senile atrophy. Bell's discovery of the functions of the anterior and posterior roots of the spinal nerves, made in 1811, was ignored in the court of final appeal in Paris, and not until 1823 was it in part accepted. Authorities disdained to recognize Dr. Bouillaud's discovery, in 1825, of the speech center of the brain, and cerebral localization of function was not appreciated until fifty years later.[4] The essay of von Helmholtz,

[1] See later discussion of opposition to Harvey, *infra*, pp. 47 *et seq*.

[2] See later discussion of opposition to Auenbrugger, *infra*, pp. 51 *et seq*.

[3] Garrison, *ibid.*, p. 360.

[4] G. M. Gould, "Reception of Medical Discoveries," *Annals of American Opthalmology*, vol. xiii, p. 722.

Uber die Erhaltung der Kraft, which later established his reputation, was first appreciated only by the mathematician, Jacobi.[1] Oliver Wendell Holmes was opposed by Hodge and Meigs, and Semmelweis by Klein, Brucke-Schmidt and other authorities, when they contended independently that puerperal fever was a contagious disease.[2]

Virchow, who had scouted the notion, in the first issue of his *Archives,* that any one man is infallible in respect to judgment and knowledge, was nevertheless later endowed with infallibility by the medical public of his day. The result was that many real advances were checked by his decisions. He declined to see anything in Charcot's ataxic joint symptoms. He held to the theory of the duality of tuberculosis. He opposed the Darwinian theory, and the new views of Behring and Koch about toxins and anti-toxins were not acceptable to him.[3] Farr and John Simon, the two greatest authorities on water-borne diseases, opposed John Snow's views that the cholera epidemic in London in 1854 was due to the Broad Street pump handle.[4] Thomas Addison's book on the ductless glands was received with incredulity and two memoirs relating similar cases not written but supported by Addison, were declined by a London Medical Society.[5] William Gull opposed surgical anaesthesia in a flippant manner,[6] and James Simpson, the chief advocate of anesthesia,[7] opposed Lister and anti-

[1] Garrison, *ibid.,* p. 572.

[2] See later discussion of opposition to the theory of puerperal fever as a contagious disease, *infra,* pp. 66 *et seq.*

[3] A. Jacobi, *Rudolph Virchow,* 1881, p. 4; Garrison, *ibid.,* p. 615.

[4] Garrison, *ibid.,* p. 801.

[5] *Dictionary of National Biography,* vol. i, p. 134.

[6] Garrison, *ibid.,* p. 678.

[7] Simpson met the opposition to anesthesia in obstetrics based on the quotation from the Bible that woman must suffer in childbirth, by indicating that the Bible relates that God caused a deep sleep to fall on Adam before the creation of Eve.

sepsis along with other authorities including Robert Lawson Tait.[1] Authorities such as Gamgee ridiculed the idea that ticks were the cause of Texas Fever.[2] Baumgarten, Emmerich and Koch opposed Metchnikoff's theory of phagocytes.[3] Patrick Manson and Dr. Carlos Finlay were sneered at by authorities because they considered mosquitoes to be disease carriers.[4] This list could be extended greatly. Gould contends that it is doubtful whether there is a single important discovery in the history of medicine which was not at first either ignored or opposed.[5] The editors of the *British Medical Journal* state emphatically, " nothing has more retarded the progress of medicine than the influence of the ' Superior Person '. To him all innovations, and especially every suggestion from the world that lies below the Olympus in the clouds of which he dwells, is heresy or even blasphemy."[6]

The conservatism of the authorities may, for the most part, be explained in terms of habit and vested interest. When one has acquired a method of investigating a certain problem, he will persistently reject an approach different from his own. Consciously and unconsciously, he selects data which substantiate prior hypotheses, and neglects to consider facts which contradict his conclusions or revaluate the phenomena or hypotheses. This is illustrated repeatedly in the instances cited above. There follows an identification of the authority with his theory which gives him a psychological vested interest in its preservation, for his reputation and pres-

---

[1] See later discussion of opposition to Lister, *infra*, pp. 80 *et seq*.
[2] Paul De Kruif, *Microbe Hunters*, 1926, p 239.
[3] Olga Metchnikoff, *Life of Elie Metchnikoff* (1921), pp. 126, 131, 148.
[4] De Kruif, *ibid.*, pp. 282, 312.
[5] Gould, *ibid.*, p. 722. See also De Kruif, *Our Medicine Men*, chap. i.
[6] *British Medical Journal*, May 27, 1911, p. 1291.

tige are involved. An economic vested interest often enters. This will be clearly illustrated in the analysis of the opposition to vaccination.

The opposition to innovations in medicine is sometimes provoked not because of the physician's inability to weigh the merits of the discovery or the " power of tradition " as expressed through the authority, but is due to the pressure of agencies outside the medical profession. Galen's teachings were so intimately bound up with church doctrine that authorities question whether Servetus' death was not primarily due to his medical concepts rather than to the theological quibble that was used as a pretext.[1] Brissot's modification of the practice of bloodletting led to his banishment by the act of Paul and Charles V in which his doctrine was denounced to be " as flagitious as Lutheranism ".[2] The effect of the church in retarding dissection and thus hindering the study of anatomy will be analyzed later.[3] Religious, political and economic factors independent of medicine suffused the vaccination controversy.[4] Samuel George Morton's teaching of the diverse origin of the races of man and the fertility of hybrids made him a target for theological hatred.[5] The opposition on the part of the church to evolution, manifested in attacks on Darwin and Haeckel, and in the fundamentalists' resistance to the teaching of evolution today, is too well

---

[1] Garrison, *ibid.*, p. 214.
[2] Garrison, *ibid.*, p. 226.
[3] See later discussion of dissection. *infra*, pp. 34 *et seq.*
[4] See later discussion of vaccination, *infra*, pp. 53 *et seq.*
[5] Kelly and Burrage, *American Medical Biographies*, 1920, p. 824; C. D. Meigs, *Memoir of S. G. Morton*, 1851, pp. 34-35. The attitude is revealed in the following contemporary quotation, " Morton's doctrines involve great moral issues, and let them be once widely circulated among the common people ... and an embroilment would result whose termination no man can foresee." Samuel D. Gross, *Lives of Eminent American Physicians and Surgeons*, 1861, pp. 595-6.

known to need extended comment.[1] Economic vested interests have consistently retarded public health movements, through their control of political machinery.[2] The cost of the antiseptic treatment and of asepsis, which retarded their use by hospitals, illustrates the role of money as a cause of inertia, a factor which frequently enters.[3]

That these influences help to prejudice physicians against certain innovations is not to be gainsaid. Medical men cannot be conceived of as scientific machines living in a void. They are subject to the same social forces as are the people among whom they live, and have religious, political and economic affiliations and prejudices.[4] They may often discount the verity of many of the objections but nevertheless be prompted by expediency to be cautious and to temper possible zealous support of an unpopular innovation. In this way other phases of culture influence the growth of medical knowledge.

Economic vested interests frequently act in opposition to the diffusion of a medical discovery through the form of propaganda of pharmaceutical concerns, who wish to retain their superseded products on the market. Suspicion is cast on the validity of the new process, and, in a skilful manner, an attempt is made to dissuade physicians from applying the

[1] For a good analysis of the opposition to Darwin, see J. Y. Simpson, *Landmarks in the Struggle between Science and Religion*, London, 1925.

[2] Garrison, *ibid.*, p. 797.

[3] See later discussion of opposition to antisepsis and asepsis, *infra*, pp. 80 *et seq.*

[4] An excellent instance of how the religious views of a medical man colored his medical opinions is the following quotation taken from Dr. Eugene Grissom's, *Medical Science in Conflict with Materialism*, 1880, pp. 2-3: "Modern society is today assailed by an insidious foe, which conceals under the guise of physiology, clothed upon by a brilliant philosophy, all the fell elements of disintegration of the whole social economy, the destruction of nobler motives of human action, the loss of the very sense of right and wrong, and the deprivation of the hope of immortality.... It is in the name of medical science that these things are boldly declared."

new method. A recent example of this procedure was the campaign against insulin.

The attitudes of medical men toward specific innovations are often complicated by their allegiance to certain cliques or factions within the profession. There has existed a historic conflict between physicians and surgeons, survivals of which one encounters today and which has been at the basis of much opposition to inventions and discoveries.[1] The tendency of the physicians influenced by the theoretical " hole-and-corner " schools of Germany in the nineteenth century " was toward wholesale contempt for the scientific achievements of men like Bichat and Magendie, Laennec and Louis, or the practical sense of such clinical workers as Bright, Stokes or Graves." [2] A conflict between research workers and practitioners results repeatedly in opposition to change. Pasteur was ignored by some because he was a chemist and not a physician.[3] Metchnikoff was snubbed by others because he was a naturalist.[4]

The personality and nationality of the innovator occasionally colors the judgment on the innovation. Purkinje was at first coldly received at Breslau on account of the current prejudice against Slavs.[5] Naunyn's rigorous Prussian manner excited much prejudice and opposition at Strassburg.[6] Pasteur's militant manner of presenting his conclusions antagonized many.[7] The personalities of Jenner and Ring in England, and Waterhouse in America aggravated the re-

[1] Garrison, *ibid.*, pp. 297-8.
[2] Garrison, *ibid.*, p. 450.
[3] Vallery-Radot, *Life of Pasteur*, pop. ed., p. 224; Paul De Kruif, *Our Medicine Men*, p. 14. See later discussion of opposition to Pasteur, p. 72.
[4] De Kruif, *Microbe Hunters*, p. 217.
[5] Garrison, *ibid.*, p. 486.
[6] Garrison, *ibid.*, p. 675.
[7] See later discussion of opposition to Pasteur, *infra*, pp. 71 *et seq.*

sistance to vaccination.¹ However, the attack on the personality of the innovator is very often a rationalization to hide the inability to refute the validity of the innovation and, as was shown above, it is often used as a device of social pressure to discourage change.

Medical education has always lagged notoriously behind the advanced practice of specialists, and in this way has contributed to medical conservatism.² An innovation must be generally accepted before it is incorporated into text books which, due to the cost involved, are not changed quickly enough to keep apace with the rapidly accumulating knowledge. The expensive apparatus requisite for the teaching of of many of the newer specialties, delay their incorporation into the curricula of the colleges. Furthermore, medical schools are exceedingly cautious in their attitude toward innovations because the prestige and reputation of the institutions are involved. This caution has been carried to such a degree that Roux was led to speak of " the tyranny of medical education ".

It is doubtful whether the masses can be called conservative in their attitude toward medical innovations. On the contrary, it is often asserted that the medical profession must be excessively cautious to counteract the tendency of the non-medical public to herald every discovery as a long sought after cure, without sufficient investigation into the claims put forward in its behalf. The masses, in their desire for relief, and in their ignorance, partly due to the deliberate secrecy surrounding medical data, are highly susceptible to all forms of medical propaganda, whether it be reactionary or progressive. The policy of the legitimate medical profession to refrain from any sort of advertising, leaves the field open to

¹ See later discussion of opposition to vaccination, *infra*, pp. 58 *et seq.*

² A. Flexner, *Medical Education in the United States and Canada*, 1910, *Medical Education in Europe*, 1912; Garrison, *ibid.*, index, Education, especially pp. 776-792.

quacks, faddists and patent medicine manufacturers to exploit the public with all sorts of "fake cures" and nostrums in which the people acquire faith on the principle of *post hoc ergo propter hoc*. Cure follows after the drug is taken, therefore it is assumed that it followed because the drug was taken, and when similar symptoms appear, it is again used. Criticisms of the medical profession by the faddists and patent medicine manufacturers with vested interests involved, is very effective and sometimes leads to opposition to a practice urged by the legitimate physicians. The psychological principle of desire to avoid pain restrains many from availing themselves of the skilled physician's services, and the factor of the size of fee sometimes prejudices them against the expert and specialist. The persistence of "folk medicines" as survivals among the masses is due to the fact that they have some utility psychologically, if not physiologically. A psychological reaction of revulsion, based on the principle of identification and intensified by ignorance, often leads to opposition on the part of the masses to certain methods employed in medical investigation such as dissection and vivisection, as will be discussed later[1] The use of "folk medicine" and recourse to faddists does not necessarily imply antagonism to the legitimate medical profession. It has correctly been said that the average American

can believe firmly and simultaneously in the therapeutic excellence of yeast, the salubrious cathartic effects of a famous mineral oil, the healing powers of chiropractors, and in the merits of the regimen of a corrective Eating Society. His catholicity of belief permits him to consider such palpable frauds seriously and at the same time to admire and respect authentic medical education and even the scientific study of disease.[2]

The man is desirous of securing relief from his ills and has

[1] See later discussion of opposition to dissection. Opposition to vivisection is considered under treatment of Pasteur, *infra,* pp. 77 *et seq.*

[2] *Civilization in the United States,* 1922, article on Medicine, p. 444.

recourse to any agency that might possibly accomplish this end. In his ignorance and because of the tendency to use the easiest and cheapest way, he sometimes rejects the advice of specialists. But his attitude toward innovations is, as a rule, very indiscriminately receptive, so much so, that he often accuses the medical profession of vested interest and jealousy because of its failure to acknowledge their value even before verification. Only when influenced by insistent adverse propaganda which exploits his medical ignorance, is he actively antagonistic.

To summarize, the present status of medicine as a science encourages conservatism. The large number of conflicting theories and methods which confront the medical man who is not equipped to verify or refute their value, force him to have recourse to authority. Authorities in medicine have, in the main, been conservative and have been prone to oppose innovations that implicate their economic and psychological vested interests and demand a reorientation of their habits of thought and practice. Medical men are also deterred from accepting innovations by religious, political and economic influences and by the propaganda of those whose vested interests are endangered. The reception of a discovery is often complicated by cliques within the profession and personality conflicts. Medical education lagging behind advanced practice, often retards change. The masses yearning for relief and cure, are undiscriminating in their support of medical innovations, a fact which has intensified the conservatism of the medical profession.

The role that psychological, cultural, mechanical and personality factors play in opposition to any particular discovery, cannot well be determined *a priori*. It can be evaluated only after a critically historical analysis has been made in each specific instance. This will be done in the following chapters in the case of examples of resistance to important progressive changes in the history of medicine.

CHAPTER III

Opposition to Dissection

DISSECTION of the human body by anatomists has met opposition, in varying degrees of intensity, from the days of the Greeks until the present. In this opposition are involved certain basic psychological reactions which are conditioned by social attitudes that are diverse in different periods and in different countries.

Antipathy to dissection can often be explained by the psychological principle of identification. The individual to whom the practice of dissection is repugnant, finds it so because he projects himself ideologically into the corpse under dissection and pictures himself being tortured with the scalpel. Horror is evoked because it is conceived that the cadaver suffers pain as would the individual who identifies himself with it. Rationalizations are then employed to hinder and, if possible, prevent the practice.

The sight of a cadaver, of corrupting flesh, or even of a skeleton often creates a revulsive physiological reaction with an accompanying gruesome emotional feeling. This is frequently followed by repugnance toward and antagonism to the dissector, probably based on the projection of this psychological state, leading to a resentment that the dissector operates on the dead body.

The social attitudes toward the "sanctity of the human body", the belief that it was impious to mutilate a form "made in the image of God", beliefs in bodily resurrection and in continued relation between the bodily remains of an individual and his "immortal spirit", the religious reverence and emotional attachment toward the deceased, and " taboos " connected with the touching of dead bodies, have determined the intensity of the reaction against dissection. The opposition, in Greek times, encountered by Herophilus and Erasistratus, may be accounted for by the hostility of the Greeks toward any interference with the bodies of the dead, and their stringent laws of the sepulchre.[1] In the Middle Ages, the dominant belief in immortality and in bodily resurrection was undoubtedly one of the factors determining the attitude of the church and the populace toward dissection. In modern times, the difference in attitude toward the dead in various countries, is reflected in their attitude toward dissection, the emphasis upon the religious and theological concepts connected with the dead body determining the intensity of opposition to a large extent.

The Bull *De sepulturis* issued by Boniface VIII in 1300, originally intended merely to prevent the practice of dismembering and boiling dead crusaders, *more teutonice,* for the purpose of more easily transporting their bodies to their native land, was enforced against dissection. This is shown by a passage in Mondino's writings and by Guido de Vigevano's introduction to his anatomical text book which stated that the church prohibited dissection.[2] The later attitudes of the Popes toward dissection were not consistently antagonistic but permission to dissect had to be obtained as an indulgence.[3] Pope Leo X, in 1519, denied Leonardo da Vinci admission to the hospital at Rome where he wished

[1] J. W. Begbie, "Early History of Anatomy," *Edinburgh Medical Journal,* 1868, vol. xiv, p. 99.

[2] Charles Singer, *Evolution of Anatomy,* p. 85 et seq.

[3] T. Puschman, *History of Medical Education,* p. 247; Georg Fischer, *Chirurgie vor 100 Jahren,* 1876, p. 94; Ed. C. Streeter, "The Role of Certain Florentines in the History of Anatomy," *Bulletin Johns Hopkins Hospital,* vol. xxvii, 1916, p. 113 et seq.

to pursue anatomical studies, because he had practiced dissection.[1]

The influence of the church in regulating dissection is brought out clearly in the description of the manner of conducting a public anatomy by Alexander Benedictus who was in Padua in the early seventeenth century.

This kind of dissection of the human body has long been permitted by Pontifical decrees; otherwise it would have been looked upon as depraved or profane. The purging of the souls of those who are to be dissected is taken care of by rites and for the indignity done unto them we make amends by prayers. For this reason many while in prison ask to be given to physicians rather than to be put to death publically at the hands of the executioner. This kind of body cannot be acquired without the Pope's consent. Lawfully, for dissecting purposes, there can be demanded lowly people and unknown persons from distant parts so that the neighborhood or relations cannot be offended. Those chosen are ones that have been suffocated by hanging. . . . Invitations are issued to the University and city officials, and when the dissection begins an introductory address sometimes preceded by music is made by the anatomist concerned. The dissection now continues from day to day until all parts are exposed. When all is done, the corpse is brought to church, followed by the clergy, the whole university and by all who had attended the anatomy, with lighted candles and finally interred by a *humanorum litterarum* professor with a long speech.[2]

The *Statua universitatis et Studii Florentini* in 1387 stipulated that mass should be said over the dissected bodies and that they should be properly buried.[3] In Paris, it was

[1] J. P. McMurrich, "Leonardo da Vinci and Vesalius," *Medical Library and Historical Journal*, Brooklyn, 1906, vol. iv, p. 344.

[2] Translated by Mortimer Frank, "Medical Instruction in the Seventeenth Century," *Journal American Medical Association*, April 24, 1915, p. 1373 *et seq.*

[3] E. C. Streeter, *Johns Hopkins Hospital Bulletin*, April, 1916, p. 113.

ordered in 1496, that the remains from dissections be buried in consecrated ground.[1]

The retardation of the practice of dissection in the Middle Ages was not due to the opposition of the Church alone, but also to the prevailing attitude toward the experimental method as a technique of the science of anatomy. The Galenic tradition had acquired an authority that was comparable only to the authority of the Church and, to question it as many dissectors did, was heresy. Charles Estienne (Stephanus—1564) who was a prominent publisher of medical books and a dissector of human bodies was persecuted, imprisoned for heresy and died in prison.

Vesalius who attacked the Galenic tradition most truculently by proof derived from human dissection was denounced violently. Sylvius called him "an impious madman whose breath poisoned Europe". Attempts were made to explain away the errors in Galen that Vesalius had revealed, by supposing a corruption of the text or by the hypothesis that the human body had changed since his time. The seven pieces of sternum which Galen had described from apes and attributed to man were interpreted as indicating how much more developed the thorax was in Galen's time; the curvature of the thigh bones, not seen in man, was said to be their natural free condition before they were straightened out by the wearing of tight breeches. The opposition to Vesalius, vehement as it was, did not culminate in a death sentence by the Inquisition as is frequently contended.[2]

[1] F. Baker, "The Two Sylviuses," *John Hopkins Hospital Bulletin*, 1909, p. 329; J. J. Walsh's *The Popes and Science* is a case of special pleading which attempts unsuccessfully to negate the importance of the influence of the Church in retarding dissection.

[2] This report is unsupported by the records of the Inquisition or of the Royal Archives. It appears to have had its origin in the letter written by Hubertus Languetus to his German friend, Kasper Peucer, dated January 8, 1565, in which he repeats the "wonderful" gossip which

In England, the practice of dissection by anatomists was retarded by the fact that the Company of Barber-Surgeons claimed exclusive monopoly rights on dissections. The following entry was made in the Annals on May 21, 1573, "Here was John Deane and appoynted to brynge in his fyne xii for havinge an Anathomye in his house contrary to an order in that behalf between this and mydsomer next".[1] In 1714, William Cheseldon, the operative surgeon at St. Thomas' Hospital was called before the court of the Barber Surgeons' Company and publicly reprimanded for the fact that he "did frequently procure the Dead Bodies of Malefactors and dissect the same at his own house contrary to the Company's by law in that behalf".[2] As late as 1745, a fine of ten pounds was imposed by the Company on any one dissecting outside of the Barber-Surgeons' Hall.[3]

The scarcity of dissection and antipathy to dissectors after the sixteenth century has been due primarily to the fact that legislation failed to provide an adequate number of cadavers to the anatomists. Tremendous pressure had always to be brought to bear upon the legislators before any advance was

had reached him alleging that Vesalius had conducted a post-mortem "on a person yet alive with heart beating." The story developed until works of high authority positively assert that Vesalius was condemned to death for this reason by the Inquisition. Andrew D. White repeated the story uncritically in his book, *The History of the Conflict between Science and Religion*. For an analysis of the report see M. Roth, *Andreas Vesalius Bruxellensis*, pp. 473-485; H. M. Spielman, *Iconography of Andreas Vesalius*, 1925, p. xiv. For a study of the work of Vesalius see in addition to Roth's book, F. H. Garrison, "In Defense of Vesalius," *Bulletin Society Medical History*, Chicago, vol. i, no. 4, pp. 47-65; F. Baker, "History of Anatomy" in *Reference Book of Medical Sciences*, vol. i, p. 329 and Charles Singer, *Evolution of Anatomy*, pp. 119 et seq.

[1] Sidney Young, *Annals of the Barber-Surgeons*, p. 317.

[2] Young, *ibid.*, p. 568.

[3] W. W. Keen, *A Sketch of the Early History of Practical Anatomy*, p. 13.

made due to the fear on their part, of the prejudice of their constituencies against dissection. This prejudice, having its roots in the psychological reactions and social attitudes mentioned above, was based also on ignorance as to the purpose of dissection, and the widespread belief that dissectors wantonly and unnecessarily mutilated dead bodies and often dissected live bodies.[1] Added to this was the fact that because the old laws only gave the bodies of legally executed murderers to the medical schools for dissection, many believed that there was something degrading in the very idea of human dissection, that it was a process to be practised only upon the bodies of the most degraded criminals.[2] The failure of the laws to provide sufficient material resulted in the practice of grave-robbing, commonly called body-snatching.

[1] The charge of dissecting live bodies made first against Herophilus and Erasistratus, and repeated against Berengar, Vesalius, Leonardo da Vinci and Michael Angelo, has recurred in all centuries as a means of inciting the people against the dissectors. A recent instance of such a specious attempt is that made by Dowie, the leader of a religious sect, in Chicago, "I could tell the story of a dissecting room where the first touch of the lancet made the supposed corpse rise from her long trance; and then as the sight burst upon her of these butchering students with their garments stained with blood, standing around her, all aghast with fear, holding their knives in their hands, she realized the horrible fact that she had been carried there for dissection, she instantly died from the shock and from the wounds inflicted by their knives.... The very best men in the profession will tell you that nineteen-twentieths of the dissections are unnecessary. But they please the devils who are preparing the doctors, and accustom the youth to the atmosphere of profanity, as they hear the filthy and unclean remarks which are made as they stand over the dead bodies and handle the sacred secrecies of humanity and laugh with diabolical glee over the consequences of a poor woman's fall or of a degraded youth's syphilitic body. I tell you this, that pollution, damnation and hell are all holding high carnival there, and a young man who escapes from that without lifelong injury is only one in a large number." J. A. Dowie, *Doctors, Drugs and Devils, or the Foes of Christ the Healer*, Zion City, Ill., 1901, pp. 20-21.

[2] To counteract this prejudice in England, Jeremy Bentham willed his body to a dissector.

This practice intensified the opposition into bitter hatred and in the popular mind dissectors were identified with violators of graves. Where the laws provided adequate dissection material to the anatomists who were therefore not obliged to have recourse to body-snatching, opposition was negligible compared to its intensity elsewhere.[1]

There were innumerable outbreaks and attacks against dissecting anatomists. In 1629, when Professor Rolfink in Jena, asked for the cadavers of criminals for dissection, the people were so wrought up that they stoned him in the street and culprits, before being executed, implored that they be not " Rolfinked ".[2] Attacks of mobs on anatomists are reported to have occurred in Lyons and Berlin in the eighteenth century provoked by the report that they were dissecting the bodies of living men.[3] Dr. William Shippen's course of anatomy lectures in Philadelphia in 1762, was interrupted repeatedly by mobs objecting to dissection, who stoned the building and threatened personal violence.[4] In 1787, the " Doctors' Mob " excited by reports concerning body-snatching, broke into the building in New York where Wright Post was teaching a course in anatomy and destroyed a valuable collection of anatomical and pathological specimens.[5] In Baltimore, a mob collected and put a forcible end to a dissection by Dr. Wiesenthal in 1788.[6] Rioters incensed

[1] *Report of Select Committee of the House of Commons on Anatomy*, London, 1828, *passim*.

[2] G. Fischer, *Chirurgie vor 100 Jahren*, p. 49.

[3] Fischer, *ibid.*, p. 95.

[4] E. M. Hartwell, " Study of Anatomy, Historically and Legally Considered," *Studies from Biological Laboratory of Johns Hopkins University*, 1883, vol. ii, p. 80.

[5] E. M. Hartwell, " Hindrances to Anatomical Studies in United States," *Annals of Anatomy and Surgery*, 1881, vol. iii, p. 229 *et seq*.

[6] E. F. Cordell, "Charles Frederich Wiesenthal," *Johns Hopkins Hospital Bulletin*, July-August, 1900, p. 170 *et seq*.

OPPOSITION TO DISSECTION

against dissectors destroyed the equipment and furniture of the college in St. Louis in 1844.[1]

Excitement ran very high against dissectors in Great Britain, especially after the exposé of the work of the " resurrectionists " in the early nineteenth century. As early as 1725, there was a public riot in Edinburgh directed against body-snatching which forced Alexander Munro to remove his anatomical preparations to greater security. On this occasion, the Incorporation of Chirurgeons published and distributed a notice deprecating and denying body-snatching and other means of obtaining bodies for dissection. It read in part, " As also the Incorporation understanding that the country people and servants in Town are frightened by a villainous report that they are in danger of being attacked and seized by Chirurgeons' apprentices in order to be dissected ". Reward was offered for information substantiating such a report.[2] In 1823, a coach drawing an empty coffin in Edinburgh was attacked by a mob and the driver was saved only by police interference. In the same year, two Americans visiting an Abbey after nightfall, were mistaken for resurrectionists and assaulted.[3] In January 1828, the detection of a body about to be exported caused a tumult in the streets of Dublin and led to the murder of a porter at the College of Surgeons.[4] The trial, in December 1828, of William Burke and William Hare, who had smothered sixteen patrons of

[1] Scharf, *History of St. Louis*, vol. ii, p. 1835, quoted by J. J. Walsh, *History of Medicine in New York*, vol. ii, p. 378.

[2] John B. Comrie, " Early Anatomical Instruction at Edinburgh," *Edinburgh Medical Journal*, vol. xxix, p. 278; John Struthers, *Historical Sketch of the Edinburgh Anatomical School*, 1867, p. 21 *et seq.*; C. H. Creswell, "Anatomy in the Early Days," *Edinburgh Medical Journal*, 1914, vol. xii, p. 149.

[3] James Blake Bailey, *The Diary of a Resurrectionist*, p. 71.

[4] C. A. Cameron, *History of the Royal College of Surgeons in Ireland*, p. 208.

their cheap boarding house and had sold their bodies to be dissected by Robert Knox, the anatomist, started a reign of terror in Edinburgh and throughout Great Britain. Knox was denounced and his life repeatedly endangered by mob attacks upon his home and lecture rooms.[1] The fact that the trial is referred to in the works of Walter Scott, DeQuincey, George Eliot, Mrs Gaskell, Robert Louis Stevenson, Charles Dickens and Robert Southey reflects the excitement created by it among the populace.[2] The trial, in London in 1831, of Bishop and Williams, who were proved to have been body-snatchers for twelve years during which time they had sold to the colleges at least five hundred bodies, raised public animosity to fever heat.[3] The excitement has gradually subsided, but is still an influence on legislation regulating dissection and is played upon by yellow journals.[4]

In opposition to dissection, one can therefore discern several psychological factors. The avoidance of pain and the unpleasant is found in the revulsion experienced at the sight of a cadaver, which, accompanied by the psychological principle of identification, results in the employment of rationalizations. It is especially difficult in the case of dis-

[1] Frank Packard, "Early British Resurrectionists," *Medical News*, July 12, 1902, pp. 64-73; A. C. Jacobson, "Robert Knox and the Resurrectionists," *Interstate Medical Journal*, vol. xxii, 1915, pp. 162-72; Bailey, *ibid., passim*.

[2] D. F. Harris, "History of Events which Led to the Passing of the Anatomy Act," *Canadian Medical Journal*, vol. x, p. 284. The word "burking" became a synonym for "smothering".

[3] Packard, *ibid.*, p. 72. This scandal led to the Warburton Act of 1832, legalizing anatomy which influenced anatomy legislation in the United States. The law was objected to by many including the editor of the *Lancet*, because it still permitted the purchase and sale of human bodies and did not create a certain source of supply. See *Lancet*, London, vol. ii, 1831-32 *passim*.

[4] *E. g.*, see bold headline of *New York Evening Journal*, April 7, 1926, reading "Chapman Grave is Hid Lest Ghouls Steal Skull for Scientist."

section, to discern whether the arguments used by the opponents are sincere, or are merely pretexts to hide the real reason for opposition, viz., the horror evoked by the practice. The opposition to the experimental method, and thus to dissection, by those who supported the Galenic tradition, was based on the tendency to suffuse a habitual mode of activity with an " emotional tone " and the persistence of habit reactions due to the difficulty of reconditioning behavior patterns. Social pressure was used against the early dissectors who opposed Galenic tradition, and by the masses of all periods against dissectors.

The cultural factors involved are: the conflict between dissection and other phases of culture, first, within the field of medicine in the form of the opposition of Galenic authority, second, with theological tenets about the " sanctity of the human body ", bodily resurrection, the relation between the body and its " immortal spirit " and taboos connected with the dead body, and third, with the attitudes of certain Popes, based on the interpretation of the Bull of Boniface VIII. This brought into play the power of established institutional authority. Vested interests motivated the activity of the Company of the Barber-Surgeons. Masses opposed dissection because of ignorance as to its purpose, and because of the belief that men were dissected alive. Mechanical difficulties of effecting change in institutional activity appear in the delay of legislatures to provide adequate dissection material.

CHAPTER IV

OPPOSITION TO HARVEY'S THEORY OF THE CIRCULATION OF THE BLOOD

THE opposition to Harvey's theory of the circulation of the blood was primarily based on the authority of tradition. Galenism was the center of the anatomists' universe in his day and it was the custom to reconcile all findings with the views of Galen. The heart was generally avoided as a field of anatomical investigation. Fracastorius held that the motion of the heart was only to be comprehended by God, and Fabricus of Aquapendente left the heart untouched in an anatomical book which appeared just prior to the publication of Harvey's work.[1] The doctrine of " spirits " held sway, substantiated by Galen's theory of heart formation, which accommodated each order of the three spirits, natural, vital and animal with its own particular workshop. To question this deeply entrenched tradition, was heresy.

Harvey realized the bold novelty of his innovation, as is shown in the dedication of his book, *De Motu Cordis,*

as this book alone declares the blood to course and revolve by a new route, very different from the ancient and beaten pathway trodden for so many ages, and illustrated by such a host of learned and distinguished men, I was afraid lest I might be charged with presumption . . . unless . . . I had confirmed its conclusions by ocular demonstrations in your presence. . . . For true philosophers, who are only eager for truth and knowledge, never regard themselves as already so thoroughly in-

[1] Willis, *Works of Harvey*, translation, London, 1847, p. 19.

formed, but that they welcome further information from whomsoever and from whencesoever it may come, nor are they so narrow-minded as to imagine any of the arts or sciences transmitted to us by the ancients, in such a state of forwardness and completion that nothing is left for the ingenuity and industry of others. . . . I profess both to learn and to teach anatomy, not from books but from dissections; not from the positions of the philosophers but from the fabric of nature.[1]

In Chapter Eight, just prior to his explanation of the circulation of the blood, he wrote,

But what remains to be said about the quantity and source of the blood which thus passes, is of so novel and unheard-of character that I not only fear injury to myself from the envy of a few, but I tremble lest I should have mankind at large for my enemies, so much doth wont and custom, that become as another nature, and doctrine once sown and that hath struck deep root, and respect for antiquity, influence all men.[2]

The effect of Harvey's teaching upon medical tradition of his time is described by a later contemporary, James De Back:

. . . by setting down the circulatory motion of the blood, innumerable axioms of ancient writers were overturned; whence it comes that all the order of teaching is troubled and the doctrine of Physick is endeavored and learned altogether preposterously and confusedly, without any certain method, which ought to be established by Positions linked together and marshalled in due order.[3]

Another later contemporary, Zachary Wood, wrote that

[1] Willis, *op. cit.*, pp. 5-7.
[2] *Ibid.*, p. 45.
[3] " *The Discourse of James De Back, physician in ordinary to the Town of Rotterdam in which he handles the nullity of spirits, Sanguification, the heat of living things—There is premised a speech to the Reader and annexed an addition in defence of Harvey's circulation,*" London, 1673.

Harvey " . . . set out a new and unheard of opinion concerning the motion of the heart and the circulation of the blood " and commented,

Truly a bold man indeed.
O disturber of the quiet of Physicians!
O seditious citizen of the Physical Commonwealth!
who first of all durst oppose an opinion confirmed for so many ages by the consent of all, and delivered up to monuments of so many Physicians, and as it were given from hand to hand to posterity, as if no man had been wise in all ages past. Indeed they do so very decently who worship antiquity as becomes them; but it is a thing unworthy in wise men who do ascribe wisdom to antiquity, with no little wrong to posterity. Therefore since to be wise, that is to say to search after truth is form with all men, they take away all wisdom from themselves who without any judgment approve of their forefathers' inventions and are by them led like cattle and do brag rashly that they see those things in them that they do not see.[1]

The reception accorded the discovery is further illustrated by a letter of Harvey written in 1649, twenty-one years after his experiments had been published.

. . . scarce a day, scarce an hour, has passed since the birthday of the circulation of the blood that I have not heard something for good or evil said of this discovery. Some abuse it as a feeble infant, and yet unworthy to have seen the light; others again think the bantling deserves to be cherished and cared for; these oppose it with much ado, those patronise it with abundant commendation; one party holds I have completely demonstrated the circulation of the blood by experiment, observation and ocular inspection, against all force and array of argument; another thinks it scarcely yet sufficiently illustrated—not yet cleared of all objections. There are some, too, who say I have

[1] Zachary Wood, physician of Rotterdam, *Preface to Harvey's Anatomical Exercises,*" 1673, pp. 2-3.

shown a vainglorious love of vivisections, and who scoff and deride the introduction of frogs and serpents, flies and others of the lower animals upon the scene, as a piece of puerile levity, not even refraining from opprobrious epithets. . . . Detractors, mummers and writers defiled with abuse, as I resolved with myself never to read them, satisfied that nothing solid or excellent, nothing but foul terms was to be expected from them, so I have held them still less worthy of an answer. . . . The authority of Galen is of such weight with all that I have seen several hesitate greatly with that experiment before them.[1]

Harvey claimed that no man over forty was found to adopt the doctrine of circulation when it was first presented.[2] At least twenty anatomists wrote against it,[3] among them Primerose,[4] Aenylius Parisanus of Venice,[5] Johannes Vesling of Padua,[6] Caspar Hoffman of Nurnburg,[7] Caecilius Folius of Venice,[8] and the elder and younger John Riolanus of Paris.[9] For the most part, the authority of Galen was evoked against him. Caspar Hoffman, who himself had rejected Galen, refused dogmatically to perform the experiment and accused Harvey of having "impeached and condemned Nature of folly and error", which attack provoked a curt

[1] Harvey's *Second Disquisition to John Riolan*, Willis edition, pp. 109-10.
[2] Willis, *Introduction to Works of Harvey*, p. xlvii.
[3] J. Donley, "Riolan and Harvey," *Annals of Medical History*, vol. v, p. 26 et seq.
[4] *Exercitationes et Animadversiones in Librum Harvei de Motu Cordis et Sanguinis*, London, 1630; see Willis, *ibid.*, p. xlii.
[5] *Lapis Lydius de Motu Cordis et Sanguinis*, Ven. 1635, Willis, *ibid.*, p. xlii.
[6] *Observationes Anatomicae et Epist. Med. ex schedis pothumis*, 1664, Willis, *ibid.* p. xliv.
[7] Willis, *ibid.*, p. xliii; D'Arcy Power, "Revised Chapter in the Life of William Harvey," *Proceedings of Royal Society of Medicine*, vol. x, Section of the History of Medicine, 1916, p. 38.
[8] Willis, *ibid.*, p. li.
[9] *Eucheiridium anatomicum et pathologicum*, 1648.

letter from Harvey. Folius based his objection on an abnormal heart condition, which he and Gassendi thought to be the normal structure and arrangement.

We learn from another source, besides the letters of Harvey quoted above, that the controversy was conducted with some heat. A contemporary, Henry Power, wrote . . .

amongst the rabble of his antagonists, we see not one that attempts to fight him at his own weapons, that is by sensible and anatomical evictions to confute that which he has by sense and autopsy so vigorously confirmed. And therefore, we cannot but look upon such scepticall and Tyrrhonian Authors as Disciples to Anaxagorous that in defiance to the noblest of his senses would needs maintain the snow was black, and shall only confute them as the walking philosopher did the Stoick, that peremptorily asserted that there was no such thing in the world as motion.[1]

The opposition of the younger John Riolanus most disturbed Harvey. He had criticised the elder Riolanus specifically in the fourth chapter of his book and seemed anxious to convince the son. Riolanus, in 1648, brought out his book on the circulation of the blood based entirely on Galen, and without the mention of a single experiment, concluding with the triumphant sentence, *" Ergo propter motum sanguinis in corde circulatorium, non est mutande Galeni methodus medendi."* [2] Harvey, in 1649, wrote two letters to Riolanus in an effort to secure his support. In 1651, he wrote to Paul Slegel of Hamburg . . .

But, perhaps, we are still to find an excuse for Riolanus, and to

[1] *Circulatio Sanguinis*, 1652, quoted by Humprey Rolleston, " The Reception of Harvey's Doctrine of the Circulation of the Blood in England as Exhibited in the Writings of Two Contemporaries " in *Essays on the History of Medicine Presented to Karl Sudhoff*, pp. 248-249.

[2] Quoted by J. Donley in " Riolan and Harvey," *Annals Medical History*, vol. v, p. 30.

OPPOSITION TO HARVEY'S THEORY

say, that what he has written is not so much of his own motion, as in discharge of the duties of his office, and with view to stand well with his colleagues. As the Dean of the College of Paris, he was bound to see the physic of Galen kept in good repair, and to admit no novelty into the school, without the most careful winnowing, lest, as he says, the precepts and dogmata of physic should be disturbed, and the pathology which has for many years obtained the sanction of the learned in assigning the causes of disease, be overthrown. He has been playing the part of the advocate, therefore, rather than of the practised anatomist.[1]

The statement of his friend, Thomas Hobbes, that Harvey was the only one in his knowledge who lived to see the new doctrine which he had promulgated victorious over opposition and established in public opinion is generally accepted.[2] There is evidence, however, that his doctrine was not so universally received and accredited, as this statement would indicate. Thomas Wiston (1575-1655) whose term of lectureship closely corresponded with Harvey's, absolutely refrains from any mention of Harvey's *De Motu Cordis*, although he frequently refers to authorities, especially to Galen, Columbus and Riolan.[3] Alexander Reid, who was the lecturer of anatomy at the Barber-Surgeons' Hall, London, published a *Manual of Anatomy* following Galen, which was reprinted six times, the last time in 1658, without an alteration in the text, recognizing Harvey's work.[4] The works of Thomas Sydenham (1624-1689) do not contain any reference to Harvey or show any conception of the significance of his discovery.[5] Descartes, in 1637, R. Drake and J. Waleaus, in 1639, H. Leroy, in 1640, G. Ent, in 1641, and Werner

---
[1] Willis, *ibid.*, p. 598.
[2] Willis, *ibid.*, p. ii; C. Singer, *Circulation of the Blood*, 1922, p. 68.
[3] Rolleston, *ibid.*, p. 250.
[4] D'Arcy Power, *Life of Harvey*, p. 231 *et seq.*
[5] Rolleston, *ibid.*, p. 250.

Rolfink, in 1641, were among those who championed the discovery.[1]

We have evidence of the effect of the opposition upon Harvey. John Aubrey writes that he had " . . . heard him (Harvey) say that after the *Circulation of the Blood* came out, he fell mightily in his practice; twas believed by the vulgar that he was crack-brained, and all the physitians were against him." That he was ridiculed and disparaged is shown by another remark of Aubrey written after the publication of Harvey's book,

though all his profession would allow him to be an excellent anatomist, I have never heard any admired his therepeutique way. I knew several practitioners in this town that would not have given three pence for one of his bills (prescriptions) and (who said) that a man could hardly tell by his bills what he did aim at.[2]

The opposition to Harvey's theory of the circulation of the blood is shown to have involved the psychological factors: first, the tendency to suffuse a habitual mode of activity with an " emotional tone ", second, fear reactions in the presence of the unknown, third, the persistence of habit reactions due to the difficulty of reconditioning behavior patterns, and fourth, the use of social pressure to exact conformity. The cultural factors were: first, the conflict between Harvey's theory and Galenic tradition which had been intimately incorporated with other phases of culture, second, the power of authority of the Galenic system, and third, ignorance as to the value of the experimental method and vivisection. Mechanical factors entered in delaying the change of text books, and curricula.

[1] Willis, *ibid.*, *passim.*
[2] Quoted by Willis, *ibid.*, p. xxiv from Aubrey, *Lives of Eminent Persons.*

CHAPTER V

RECEPTION OF AUENBRUGGER'S THEORY OF PERCUSSION

LEOPOLD AUENBRUGGER, in 1761, made public his epoch-making discovery of the use of immediate percussion of the chest in diagnosis, based upon observation verified by post mortem experiences and experiment. In the preface to his book he wrote,

In making public my discoveries respecting this matter, I have been actuated neither by an itch for writing nor a fondness for speculation but by the desire of submitting to my brethren the fruits of seven years observation and reflection. In doing so, I have not been unconscious of the dangers I must encounter, since it has always been the fate of those who have illustrated or improved the arts and sciences by their discoveries to be beset by envy, malice, hatred, detraction and calumny.[1]

He met the treatment he had anticipated in the hands of those who upheld the established tradition. Van Swieten, his teacher, made no mention of his book, in his discussion of the diseases of the chest which appeared in 1761. De Haen did not mention percussion in his eighteen-volume *Ratio Medendi*. Vogel of Göttingen, whose opinion was authoritative at that time, evidently had not read Auenbrugger's book, for he regarded percussion as an imitation of Hippocrates' succussion. Sprengel, Baldinger and other contemporary writers, also snubbed the innovation. Peter Frank gave it but a frosty commendation, and only Haller, Stoll, Ludwig, and Roziere of Montpellier, who translated it into French,

---

[1] *Inventum Novum*, 1761, see translation in Camac's *Epoch Making Contributions to Medicine, Surgery and Allied Sciences*, 1909, p. 123.

were friendly in Auenbrugger's lifetime. The work was slighted and ignored and remained practically unknown until Corisart's authority, in 1808, secured its recognition.[1] Even as late as 1840, Wolff in Berlin conducted a *lateinische Klinik* where there was neither percussion nor auscultation.[2]

The slowness of the diffusion of Auenbrugger's discovery may be attributed to two main causes. In the first place, the profession of his time devoted itself primarily to the study of the Hippocratic doctrines and their elaboration, and were not animated by the desire to enlarge the boundaries of medical science by experiment and investigation. Experimental studies such as those of Auenbrugger were therefore disdained. In the second place, Auenbrugger was never a teacher and therefore had no pupils who might learn and extend his discovery among the profession.[3]

The psychological factors involved in delaying the diffusion of Auenbrugger's discovery of percussion were the tendency to suffuse an habitual mode of activity with an "emotional tone" and the persistence of habit due to the difficulty of reconditioning behavior patterns. The cultural factors were: conflict with the established practices, ignorance of the value of the experimental method, and the power of authority. The mechanical factor of the difficulty of diffusing knowledge appears prominently in this instance.

[1] Max Neuburger, *Leopold Auenbrugger*, Vienna, 1922; S. Weir Mitchell, "The Early History of Instrumental Precision in Medicine," *Transactions Congress American Physicians*, New Haven, 1891, vol. ii, p. 180; *British Medical Journal*, London, 1909, vol. i, p. 1191; Edgar P. Copeland, "Leopold Auenbrugger," *Virginia Medical Semi-Monthly*, 1914, vol. xix, p. 94; Garrison, *op. cit.*, p. 363.

[2] Garrison, *ibid.*, p. 778.

[3] E. O. Otis, "Auenbrugger and Laennec," *Boston Medical and Surgical Journal*, vol. 139, Sept. 22, 1898, p. 283.

CHAPTER VI

THE OPPOSITION TO VACCINATION [1]

THE history of the vaccination controversy illustrates opposition to the diffusion of a medical innovation in which many of the factors which enter into opposition to social change are involved. These factors are intimately bound up with one another but can be isolated and discussed individually. The causes of the original resistance of certain individuals in the medical profession to the innovation will first be considered and then the basis of the popular opposition to vaccination, which has assumed tremendous proportions in different countries from the introduction of the practice to the present day.

Vested interests in the medical profession manifested themselves in opposition to vaccination immediately upon its introduction by Jenner in 1798. The practice of inoculating with small pox virus, called variolation, was a specialty among certain physicians who derived their entire income from this source. The large majority of the early opponents to vaccination were of the group of specialists whose financial interests were threatened. Joseph Merry,[2] John Frank,[3]

---

[1] For a detailed historical and critical investigation of the opposition to vaccination see the author's book, *Should We Be Vaccinated: A Survey of the Controversy in its Historical and Scientific Aspects*, Harper and Brothers, 1927.

[2] *A Conscious View of Circumstances and Proceedings Respecting Vaccine Innoculation.*

[3] *Medical and Physical Journal*, vol. iv, 1800, p. 521.

Birch,[1] Rowley,[2] Squirell,[3] Lipscomb,[4] Shillito,[5] Rogers,[6] all were small pox inoculators, who through their publications sought to discredit the new method and retain their practices. Moseley, who was the outstanding figure in the early opposition movement, exploited the interest in the vaccination question to secure publicity for " Dr. Moseley's Pills ".[7] From the beginning of the controversy until the present, medical faddists have participated actively in anti-vaccination campaigns. As John Simon expressed it " . . . quacks with their touters have often found it convenient to hitch themselves on the skirts of a discussion in which the public has been interested, ready for any chance of reviling the science which condemns their wretched arts; but above all, eager to

[1] *Letter Occasioned by Many Failures of Cow Pox*, 1804; *Serious Reasons for Uniformly Objecting to the Practice of Vaccination*, 1806.

[2] *Cow Pox Innoculation No Security Against Small Pox Infection, with above five hundred proofs of failure. To which are added the modes of treating the beastly new diseases produced from cow pox. Explained by two coloured copper plate engravings, and five hundred dreadful cases of small pox after vaccination or Cow-Pox Mange, Cow-Pox Ulcers, Cow-Pox Evil or Abscess, Cow-Pox Mortification. With the author's certain experienced and successful mode of Innoculating for small pox which now becomes necessary from cow-pox failure*, 1805.

[3] *Observations addressed to the public in general on the cow pox shewing that it originates in Scrophula commonly called the evil; Illustrated with cases to prove that it is no security against the Small Pox. Also pointing out the dreadful consequences of the new Disease so recently introduced into the Human Constitution. To which are added Observations on the Small Pox Innoculation, proving it to be more beneficial to society than the Vaccine*, 1805.

[4] *Dissertations on the Failure and Mischiefs of the Disease of Cow Pox*, 1805; *Cow Pox Exploded, or the Inconsistencies Absurdities and Falsehoods of Some of its Defenders Exposed*, 1806; *Innoculation for the Small Pox Vindicated*, 1805.

[5] *Cases of Cow Pox Failures and Mischiefs*, 1808.

[6] *Examination of Cow Pox Evidence*, 1805.

[7] *Medical Tracts*, 1799; *Treatise on Lues Bovilla*, 1805; *Review of Report of the Royal College of Physicians on Vaccination*, 1808.

assure their dupes that while vaccination is so worthless a precaution, life may be prolonged and youth made perpetual by one incomparable pill or elixir ".[1] Patent medicine manufacturers, osteopaths, chiropractors, hydropaths, Christian Scientists, naturopaths and other such sectarian groups have been the outstanding proponents and financial supporters of the recent anti-vaccination movement.

The arguments used by the early anti-vaccinationists with vested economic interests involved were manifestly not sincere. They were concerned with discrediting vaccination and sought to do so not only on the basis of possibly valid criticism of the original overstatements of its effectiveness, but by exploiting the medical ignorance of the masses of people by creating fear, repulsion and aversion to the innovation. It is certainly doubtful that Rowley and Moseley believed that cow-pox inoculation brought with it the diseases they described as being the result of the " bestial humour ". One cannot determine this definitely because the knowledge of the causes of epidemic diseases and immunity was entirely lacking at that time, and even John Sims, the president of the London Medical Society, who afterward became an advocate of vaccination, at first questioned whether the " infection by an inoculation of a variety of acrid animal poisons " would not introduce new diseases.[2] Furthermore, the limitation of the scientific medical equipment of Moseley is shown by the fact that he believed the phases of the moon to be a cause of hemorrhage of the lungs.[3] Yet the use of engravings to show how children who had been vaccinated were developing cow's faces, and the description of " Cow-pox Mange ", " Cow Pox Ulcers ", " Cow Pox Evil or Abscess " and " Cow Pox Mortification " by Rowley [4] and

[1] British Royal Commission on Vaccination, Final Report, 1889, p. 71.
[2] *Medical and Physical Journal*, vol. i, 1799, p. 11.
[3] *Dictionary of National Biography*, article, Benj. Moseley.
[4] Rowley, *op. cit., passim.*

by Moseley of "Facies Bovilla or Cow Pox Face", "Scabies Bovilla or Cow Pox Itch or Mange", "Tinea Bovilla or Cow Pox Scaldhead", and "Elephantiasis Bovilla or Cow Pox Farcy"[1] have the appearance not of ignorant, mistaken judgments but of unscrupulous attempts to frighten the masses away from vaccination. The same is true of the writings of the other inoculators mentioned above, as well as those in other countries who never failed to urge variolation after condemning vaccination in violent abusive language and describing its resultant horrors in graphic detail.

Various other devices were employed by these men in opposing the practice. They portrayed Jenner and other vaccinationists as making fortunes on a worthless procedure; they argued that if vaccination were really a prophylactic against small pox, physicians would not adopt it because they make money on the ills of people and it would therefore lower their income.[2] Rivalries between communities and hatred for anything French on the part of the English populace were all skillfully exploited by the anti-vaccinationists.[3] Malthus' population theory, then in vogue among the conservatives in England, was used against it.[4]

Since vaccination has become the established practice, the argument of vested interest has been used repeatedly by the anti-vaccinationists to discredit the advocacy of physicians and public health officers of its efficacy. This is the leading argument of George Bernard Shaw, whose anti-vaccination activity is only one phase of his attack on the medical profession as a "trust"[5] and of all the medical sectarians and

[1] *Treatise on Lues Bovilla*, 2nd ed., p. 105.
[2] *E. g.*, Merry, *op. cit., passim.*
[3] *Medical Observer*, March, 1808, vol. ii, p. 170.
[4] J. Birch, *Serious Reasons, etc.*, p. 28.
[5] Preface to *The Doctor's Dilemma*, 1906; Statement in 1912 quoted in the *Jennerian*, June 15, 1912, p. 34; Preface to *Back to Methuselah*, 1921, p. 13.

faddists.[1] The attack loses its convincing tone in the light of the inquiries into the vaccination question, the most intensive of which were those in England in 1802, 1807 and 1889-1896, in Denmark in 1804, in Germany in 1882, and in Pennsylvania in 1913, all of which emphatically endorsed the practice. In fact, in order to protect their financial interests, many physicians in the United States have opposed " state medicine " and have therefore interfered with state control of vaccination.

The vehement enthusiasm with which the theory of vaccination was promulgated in England by Jenner, Pearson, Woodville and Ring, and the tremendous influence of the authority of Lettsom who supported the innovation, caused vaccination to receive early acceptance among the leading physicians in England after the substantiating evidence presented by Pearson and Woodville, in spite of the novelty of the procedure and the " power of tradition ". This can partly be explained by the great need of a prophylactic against small pox at that time, and the relative simplicity of the operation. There was, however, less ready acceptance in America where Waterhouse in Boston spoke of the " chilling apathy and repellent suspicion " with which his plans were received, and Seaman in New York, Coxe, Rush, Oliver and Currie in Philadelphia and James Smith of Baltimore all complained of the antagonism to the practice on the part of the rest of the profession. In Germany, Stromeyer of Hanover stated in 1800 that " most of our physicians here exclaim against the vaccine inoculation ",[2] and Dr. Stuve of Gorlits wrote in 1802 that " . . . calumniators were not wanting who vented their spleen against me as a vaccinator; for many persons were my enemies on that account and

[1] *E. g.* Robert A. Gunn, *Vaccination, Its Fallacies and Evils*, 1882, p. 29.
[2] Letter to the *Medical and Physical Journal*, vol. iii, p. 471.

almost everyone was envious ",[1] but the practice seems nevertheless to have diffused comparatively rapidly. In France too, in spite of the propaganda of the small pox inoculators, vaccination was received by the profession with little opposition. The loud and clamorous opposition in all countries of the small groups whose vested interests were involved received tremendous response among the laity for reasons which will be discussed later.

Much of the opposition that arose after vaccination had been practiced for a number of years was due to the fact that Jenner and his followers made excessive claims for vaccination, on the ground that it gave permanent immunity against small pox. The valid opposition, in all countries, on the part of those who did not reject vaccination *in toto,* but who urged revaccination [2] was also exploited by those who had vested interests involved. In this phase of the controversy, it was the proponents of vaccination who were conservative. They did not desire to acknowledge that only temporary relief was afforded and to demand revaccination, lest it cast discredit upon their earlier assertions and thus upon vaccination. Many years passed, therefore, before revaccination was urged as being necessary. It must also be acknowledged that the careless manner in which vaccination was performed for many years after its introduction undoubtedly led in many cases to other complications and therefore merited some of the criticism leveled against it. The precautions taken today obviate such dangers.

Personality conflicts colored the controversy. Jenner's hypersensitive and self-conscious nature which led to a militantly aggressive attack on all who differed from him in the slightest detail, irritated many who wished to approach the

[1] Ring, *A Roland for an Oliver,* 1807, p. 91.

[2] See particularly William Goldson, *Cases of Small Pox Subsequent to Vaccination,* 1804, and Thomas Brown, *An Inquiry into the Antivariolous Power of Vaccination,* 1809.

question of vaccination with more scientific calm. Jenner's desire to be the sole recipient of the honor of introducing vaccination to the world, led to unjustifiable attempts to detract from the work of Pearson and Woodville, whose corroborative evidence had established the practice. This resulted in bitter partisanship between them. These altercations and the quarrels between Ring and Walker, both pro-vaccinationists, gave the anti-vaccinationists opportunity to disparage the work of the vaccinationists. Maclean's anti-vaccination activity was also due to a personality conflict provoked by his personal antagonism to Lucas Pepys who was in charge of the National Vaccine Establishment.

The controversial personality and religious and political affiliations of Benjamin Waterhouse, who introduced vaccination into the United States, contributed to the extreme opposition to the innovation in Massachusetts. His professional associates resented the airs which he assumed due to his scientific training abroad, and were decidedly antagonistic to him. Added to this, the fact that he was a dissenter belonging to the sect of Friends, and a Jeffersonian Republican at odds with the aristocratic group of Federalists that controlled affairs in Boston, intensified the opposition vaccination encountered under his sponsorship.[1]

The devices to exact conformity to the traditional procedure were used profusely when vaccination was first introduced. Ridicule was the chief weapon of the opponents. They accused the proponents of vaccination as being victims of " cow-mania ", sneered at the method of preventing small pox which Jenner had learned from dairy maids, and caricatured the personal eccentricities of the leading vaccinators.[2]

[1] Kelly and Burrage, *American Medical Biographies*, article, Benjamin Waterhouse, p. 1202; F. Packard, *History of Medicine in America*, 1901, p. 231.

[2] See any of the works of Benj. Moseley, especially, *An Oliver for a Rowland*, which was a scurrilous, salacious attack on Roland Hill. Also see the periodical, *The Cow Pox Chronicle*.

The latter were kept always on the defensive by repeated charges of failures, and by the claim that they were introducing new diseases. These tactics were only effective with the timid in the medical profession until the leading physicians endorsed the practice, but they had far-reaching results among the laity.

Apart from the temporary hesitancy on the part of the medical profession to accept Jenner's conclusions which were based on insufficient data until corroborated by the work of Pearson and Woodville and endorsed by Lettsom, the opposition to vaccination was confined therefore to those whose vested interests were involved through the decline of the practice of variolation, and Moseley, whose activity was due partly to ignorance which made him fear the dangers of the innovation and partly to the fact that he profited financially by his continued opposition. The medical profession, since its first acceptance of the principle, has never doubted the efficacy of the practice although it has modified the procedure with more precautionary methods and has found revaccination to be a necessary additional protection. An anti-vaccination campaign has, however, been part of the tactics of every medical sect, who exploit the public's persistent opposition to vaccination. The causes of this resistance of the laity to vaccination will now be considered.

At the basis of much of the opposition to vaccination by the laity lies the psychological principle of desire to avoid pain. No matter how skillful the operation, it always involves discomfiture from which the individual shrinks. Ashamed of this cowardice, he uses rationalizations which would justify his not being vaccinated. These rationalizations can be divided roughly into two types, those that would discount the efficacy of vaccination and emphasize its dangers and those that would attack vaccination on religious and political grounds.

It is manifestly difficult for the laity, ignorant as it is of scientific medicine, to deal adequately with the medical and statistical factors involved in the proof that vaccination is an effective preventive from small pox. People are aware of the fact that small pox, once a most dreaded disease, is now practically eliminated but it is easy to question as to whether this fact can be ascribed to vaccination. They have heard of cases of small pox after vaccination and are sceptical of the physician's explanation of this phenomenon. They do not comprehend the variations in degree of immunity nor the reasons for the physician's insistence on repeated revaccination, which often seems to them a refusal to admit failure. The fact that in every small-pox epidemic, it has been the unvaccinated who succumb in an overwhelmingly greater number, is either unknown, ignored or discounted in the desire to select evidence that substantiates their rationalization. It is also now urged as an excuse that since small pox has become rare, vaccination and revaccination are unnecessary precautions.

The danger which vaccination carries with it is given exaggerated importance because the experience with one unfortunate case outweighs, in intensity of impression, any number of successful operations. Such unfortunate cases comprise a negligible, almost infinitesimal number compared to those cases where no complications develop but there still remains that fear of possible danger, and the individual in his desire to avoid pain is timorous. This fear is intensified by the vivid and gruesome emphasis of the anti-vaccinationists on these dangers. Since vaccination was first introduced, the supposed horrible consequences of vaccination have been described in a lurid manner, the increase of every disease known has been ascribed to vaccination, and the danger of being infected with syphilis has been especially stressed.[1]

[1] *E. g.* John Gibbs, *Compulsory Vaccination*, 1856; Bayard, *Influence de la Vaccine sur la Population*, 1856; Verde-Delisle, *De la degenerescence physique et morale de l'espece humaine determine par le Vaccin*, 1855; Tracts of the New York Anti-Vaccination Society, 1926.

The characterization of cow-pox lymph by the anti-vaccinationists as "acrid animal poison derived from diseased brutes", also created apprehension among the ignorant.

It is not surprising that as a result of this propaganda, the masses dread vaccination. The medical theories discrediting vaccination are given far greater publicity than the facts that substantiate the practice, and many are therefore confused and frightened. Unable to weigh the facts or even the validity of the authority that challenges the practice, they are prone to avoid pain and possible danger, by not being vaccinated. The physician's endorsement of vaccination is often seriously questioned since he is an interested party because of the fees which he derives through vaccination.

The argument that better sanitation and better living conditions are responsible for the decline of the small-pox rate and not vaccination, has had great appeal to the masses, especially among the exploited poor who are fighting for improved living conditions. To them, vaccination is merely palliative, the more fundamental problem being the effacement of the poverty and wretchedness resulting from the present maldistribution of wealth. The necessity of eliminating the causes which breed and make men susceptible to diseases is stressed rather than the value of immunizing people against them. This program is of fundamental importance, but it does not negate the value and necessity of vaccination under present conditions. The British Royal Commission, furthermore, showed conclusively that although sanitation undoubtedly had an influence upon the decreasing rate of incidence and mortality of small pox, yet there was not enough variation in the sanitary conditions in the first quarter of the eighteenth century as compared to that of the last half of the seventeenth century to account for the decrease, and that if improved sanitary conditions were the cause, they would have exercised a similar influence over measles, scarlet fever, whooping cough and other diseases spread by contagion and infection, instead of only in the case of small pox where the additional factor of vaccination was present.[1] The sanitation argument, however, has been the most persuasive attack on vaccination. To some it is a program of social reform; to others, it merely affords another rationalization to avoid the personal pain and possible danger of vaccination.

The attempt of the masses to avoid vaccination on the religious grounds that it was " sinful and doubting of Providence " was prevalent in all countries when vaccination was first introduced and it persisted for many years.[2] It was argued that to immunize oneself against small pox by vaccination was to attempt to interfere with " the plans of God ". The writers whose vested interests were involved, always stressed this popular rationalization and the early proponents of vaccination found it especially necessary to secure the cooperation of the clergy in an attempt to dispel the concept.

When vaccination became compulsory the attack on the grounds that it was an interference with personal liberty eclipsed all others. The attempt at enforcement of the practice on those who resisted vaccination for medical or religious reasons led to punishment of the objectors with the resulting resentment of many who believed in vaccination but not in its compulsory enforcement. In England, especially, has there been vehement objection to compulsory vaccination on the basis of the belief in the tradition of personal liberty. Herbert Spencer, consistent with his belief in the non-interference of the state in individual freedom expressed himself against vaccination.[3] Alfred Russel Wallace joined the con-

[1] British Royal Vaccination Commission, Final Report, 1896, pp. 18-19, 39-46.

[2] Wm. Lovett, *Life and Struggles*, Knopf ed., vol. i, p. 5; John Daglish, *Practical Observations on Vaccine Inoculation*, 1825, p. 29.

[3] *Social Statics*, pp. 212-13.

troversy aroused by the imprisonment and fining of those who refused to be vaccinated.[1] John Bright, although in favor of vaccination considered its compulsory enforcement unwise.[2] The objection to compulsory vaccination became so insistent that it led to the investigation of the British Royal Commission on Vaccination of 1889-1896, which reported that

. . . When that which the law enjoins runs counter to the convictions or prejudices of many members of the community, it is not easy to secure obedience to it. And when it imposed a duty on parents the performance of which they, honestly, however erroneously, regard as seriously prejudicial to their children, the very attempt to compel obedience may defeat the object of the legislation.[3]

Their recommendation to recognize the "conscientious objector" was passed by Parliament in 1898, and the act of making the declaration of objection was made easier in 1907. The fact that the protest against compulsion was on the part of most individuals prompted by a desire to avoid vaccination is shown by the extraordinarily large number of exemptions requested.[4]

In summarizing, the factors involved in the opposition of the medical profession during the early stages of the vaccination controversy, must be distinguished from those causing the opposition of the masses. The psychological factors at the basis of the former were first, the tendency to suffuse an habitual mode of activity with an emotional tone; second

---

[1] British Royal Commission on Vaccination, Third Report, 1890, p. 127. His book, *Vaccination a Delusion, its Penal Enforcement a Crime*, had a very large circulation.

[2] British Royal Commission on Vaccination, Third Report, 1890, p. 114.

[3] British Royal Commission on Vaccination, Final Report, 1896, p. 137.

[4] British Ministry of Health, *Small Pox and Vaccination*, 1921, p. 12.

fear in the presence of the unknown; third, the persistence of habit reactions due to the difficulty of reconditioning behavior patterns; fourth, the mechanism of rationalization; fifth, the use of social pressure to exact conformity. The cultural factors were first, the vested interests of the inoculators; second, the ignorance of the principle of immunity on the part of the medical profession when vaccination was first introduced; third, the conflict between vaccination and the established practice of inoculation. The personality factor was involved in England because of Jenner and in America because of Waterhouse.

In the opposition of the masses, there were the psychological factors: first, the avoidance of pain and the unpleasant; second, fear; and third, the use of rationalizations. The cultural factors were first, the conflict between vaccination and other phases of culture (a) in that its enforcement was considered futile and dangerous by those who held that sanitation was the cause of the decline of the small-pox rate, (b) in the form of conflict between state medical control, made necessary by vaccination, and the political ideal of individual liberty; (c) in the clash of vaccination with certain religious concepts. Ignorance has been the cultural factor which has exaggerated the fear of the danger resulting from vaccination. The mechanical difficulties of diffusing knowledge and of legislative action are also prominent in the case of vaccination.

CHAPTER VII

OPPOSITION TO HOLMES AND SEMMELWEIS

OLIVER WENDELL HOLMES in America and Ignaz Semmelweis in Vienna, who independently propounded the theory that puerperal fever was a contagious disease often carried by surgeons, both met strenuous opposition on the part of the established authorities of their period.

Oliver Wendell Holmes' article first appeared in April 1843, in the *New England Quarterly Journal of Medicine and Surgery,* when he was thirty-four years old and held no university position. Little attention was paid to it until 1852 and 1854, when Meigs, professor of midwifery at the Jefferson Medical College, Philadelphia, and Hodge, professor of obstetrics at the University of Pennsylvania, both prominent authorities, attacked the theory. They attributed puerperal fever to " chance or Providence ", and denied vigorously that they were ever the vehicle of transmission of the disease. Holmes republished the essay in 1855, as professor of anatomy at the Harvard Medical School, prefacing it with a vehement introduction portraying the controversy. It concluded,

. . . this is no subject to be smoothed over by nicely adjusted phrases of half assent and half censure divided between the parties. The balance must be struck boldly and the result declared plainly . . . persons are nothing in this matter, better that twenty pamphleteers should be silenced or as many professors unseated, than that one mother's life should be taken. There is no quarrel here between men but there is deadly incompatibility and exterminating warfare between doctrines. . . . If I am wrong, let me be put down by such a rebuke as no rash disclaimer has received since there has been a public opinion in the medical profession of America; if I am right, let doctrines which lead to professional homicide be no longer taught from the chairs of those two great Institutions. Indifference will not do here; our journalists and committees will have no right to take up their pages with minute anatomy, and tediously detailed cases while it is a question whether or not the 'black death of child bed' be scattered broadcast by the agency of the mother's friend and advisor. Let the men who mould opinions look to it; if there is any voluntary blindness, any interested oversight, any culpable negligence, even, in such a matter, and the facts shall reach the public ear; the pestilence carrier of the lying-in chamber must look to God for pardon for men will never forgive him.[1]

The opposition to Semmelweis was even more acrimonious. The novelty of the innovation aroused strenuous objection.

It had to be confessed that all that had been taught for years about which thick-bellied books full of learning had been written, was error throughout; that a small piece of chloride of lime was sufficient to throw upon the scrap heap the whole learned apparatus which so many distinguished men of science had been collecting and elaborating for centuries, with the industry and perseverance of bees; that the application of chloride of lime was sufficient to arrest an outbreak of the disease against which all efforts had hitherto been put forth in vain. All that appeared to be too simple to be seriously accepted.[2]

Puerperal fever continued to be explained in terms of atmospheric, cosmic, telluric influences.

The authority of Virchow militated against the acceptance of the doctrine. He did not attack it in any way but treated it with disdainful silence while teaching the conflicting

[1] Camac, *Epoch Making Contributions to Medicine and Surgery*, p. 397.
[2] William Sinclair, *Life of Semmelweis*, p. 111.

theories. When Semmelweis attacked the views of Virchow, he was denounced for his temerity.[1]

Personality conflicts intensified the controversy. Semmelweis, who is characterized as " irascible, impatient and tactless "[2] finally went insane and committed suicide because of the treatment accorded him.[3] His act of enrolling in the " academic Legion ", a revolutionary force formed as a result of the rejection of a petition of the Diet of Lower Austria by Emperor Ferdinand, incurred the antagonism of the reactionary Klein, who, therefore, did not reappoint him as his assistant.[4] Skoda's blunt advocacy of Semmelweis' doctrine aroused additional opposition. Scanzoni of Prague, considered the frank expressions of adverse opinion contained in Skoda's address to be a personal attack and proceeded to publish a vindication.[5] The opposition of Carl Braun, Klein's successor, was also largely personal. When he was appointed as assistant in Semmelweis' place, he repeatedly referred to the doctrine of his predecessor as all " humbug ". When it was pointed out to him that from the very month in which he himself commenced work at the Lying-in Hospital, the mortality began to rise and went on increasing during the year and one-half before Semmelweis left Vienna, Braun became a personal antagonist of Semmelweis.[6]

Semmelweis' work was for the most part ignored. A commission appointed in Prague in 1849 at Scanzoni's suggestion to inquire into the whole question of puerperal fever, of which Hamernik was a member, had not made a report in 1860.[7] The result was that when Lister visited the

[1] Sinclair, *ibid.*, p. 168.
[2] *Encyclopedia Brittanica*, 11th ed., vol. xxiv, p. 631, article Ignaz Semmelweis.
[3] Garrison, *ibid.*, p. 459.
[4] Sinclair, *ibid.*, pp. 72, 112.
[5] Sinclair, *ibid.*, pp. 62, 93.
[6] Sinclair, *ibid.*, pp. 155-6.
[7] Sinclair, *ibid.*, pp. 94, 262.

continent in 1883, the name of Semmelweis was not even mentioned.[1]

Much of the opposition to Semmelweis was based on a misunderstanding of his teaching, the belief that he ascribed cadaveric poison as the sole cause of puerperal fever. He was called " the apostle of cadaveric poison, the preacher of a one-sided creed " although in an address delivered before the Vienna Medical Society in 1850, he made plain that this was not his doctrine.[2]

The device of malignant ridicule was employed against Semmelweis.[3] Surgeons used sarcasm when referring to him as a physician who expressed opinions upon surgical questions which were outside his province.[4] When Weigert attempted to make Semmelweis' work known in France, his article was published in the *Union Medicale* under the heading of " doubtful anecdotes ".[5] The question of priority also arose in the attempt to discredit Semmelweis. Zipfel who first congratulated Semmelweis, confiding that he had very nearly made the discovery himself, later claimed that he and Fergusson were the discoverers of the true cause of puerperal fever.[6]

To summarize, the " power of tradition ", both in the instance of Holmes and Semmelweis, made it difficult for the theory of puerperal fever as a contagious disease to secure recognition, especially since authorities for the most part ignored the innovation or rejected it because it accused surgeons of being carriers of disease, a charge which had to be denied for self-defense. Personality conflicts in the case

---

[1] *Encyclopedia Brittanica*, 11th ed., vol. xvi, p. 779.
[2] Sinclair, *ibid.*, pp. 87, 101, 234.
[3] Sinclair, *ibid.*, p. 63.
[4] Sinclair, *ibid.*, p. 84.
[5] Sinclair, *ibid.*, p. 100.
[6] Sinclair, *ibid.*, p. 102.

of Semmelweis augmented the opposition. The devices of social pressure, ridicule, indifference, deliberate misinterpretation, and attempts to discredit on the basis of priority, all were used against Semmelweis in an attempt to discourage deviation from the established tradition. Psychological vested interests and the difficulty of reconditioning behavior patterns were the psychological factors, and ignorance was the cultural factor underlying the opposition.

CHAPTER VIII

Opposition to Pasteur and His Discoveries

THE controversies that ensued following Pasteur's announcement of his discoveries illustrate effectively many of the factors that enter to prevent the diffusion of innovations. The causes which provoked opposition to Pasteur vary in the case of each of the discoveries, yet upon analysis certain of them are shown to be constant.

One who reads the *Life of Pasteur* by his son-in-law, Vallery-Radot, will discern, even in spite of the highly laudatory and eulogistic tone of the work, that Pasteur's personality was one that aroused antagonism by its violent aggressiveness and cocksureness. De Kruif's excellent characterization of Pasteur bears out the thought that this had much to do with the opposition he always encountered,

Pasteur made these enemies not entirely because his discoveries stepped on the toes of old theories and beliefs. No, his bristling, curious, impudent air of challenge got him enemies. He had a way of putting "am - I - not - clever - to - have - found - this - and - aren't - all - of - you - fools - not - to - believe - it - at - once", between the lines of all his writings and speeches. He loved to fight with words, he had cocky eagerness to get into an argument with every one about anything. He would have sputtered indignantly at an innocently intended comment on his grammar or his punctuation.[1]

Dr. Jules Guerin felt called upon to rebuke him on one instance at the Academy of Medicine because of his boast-

---
[1] Paul De Kruif, *Microbe Hunters*, p. 74.

fulness,[1] and a professor at Turin was provoked to publish a little pamphlet entitled *The Scientific Dogmatism of the Illustrious Professor Pasteur*.[2] Pasteur's personal unpopularity is also indicated by the fact that in 1873 he was elected to the vacancy in the Free Association of the Academy of Medicine by a majority of only one vote although he had been first on the section's list.[3]

The fact that Pasteur was a laboratory chemist and not a practising physician, influenced many medical men against his discoveries. The dicta of the surgeon Chassaignac to Pasteur typify this attitude: " Laboratory results should be brought out in a circumspect, modest and reserved manner, so long as they have not been sanctioned by long clinical researches, a sanction without which, there is no real and practised medical science ". He then proceeded to denounce the idea of bacteria as cause of disease.[4] The distrust felt by the physicians for chemists was a long-standing tradition in France. Vallery-Radot quotes a statement from the *Traite de Therapeutique* published in 1855 by Trousseau and Pidoux:

When the chemist has seen the chemical conditions of respiration, of digestion, or of the action of some drug, he thinks he has given the theory of those functions and phenomena. It is ever the same delusion which chemists will never get over. We must make up our minds to that, but let us beware trying to profit by the precious researches which they would probably never undertake if they were not stimulated by the ambition of explaining what is outside their range.[5]

[1] Vallery-Radot, *The Life of Pasteur*, p. 309.
[2] Vallery-Radot, *ibid.*, p. 372.
[3] Vallery-Radot, *ibid.*, p. 225.
[4] Vallery-Radot, *ibid.*, p. 228.
[5] Vallery-Radot, *ibid.*, p. 224.

Many silkworm cultivators criticized the Government for choosing a "mere chemist" to study the disease that was destroying the silk industry of France instead of some zoologist or silk-worm cultivator.[1]

The "power of tradition" manifests itself as a factor in all instances of opposition to Pasteur's discoveries. It is not surprising that theories as novel as his should be received sceptically. The great authorities, Liebig and even Helmholtz [2] could be quoted against Pasteur and therefore retarded the acceptance of the theory of fermentation for many years.[3] Liebig was especially conservative. He refused to believe that yeast is alive and declined to look through a microscope.[4] Although in 1836, Cagniard Latour and Schwann independently had reported on the organic nature of yeast, M. Dumas and Claude Bernard in 1850 spoke of the act of fermentation as "strange and obscure".[5] Pasteur's experiments involving as they did data and reasoning which were unfamiliar to many men and resulting in conclusions contrary to authority were therefore accepted hesitatingly.

Pasteur's rejection of spontaneous generation and his contention, in De Kruif's phraseology, that "microbes must have parents" ran counter to the established current tradition of his day. Joly and Musset, and Pouchet were at first not convinced by Pasteur's experiments and demanded a commission to test them. The controversy was conducted with some heat. Joly was applauded when he declared at a lecture before the Faculty of Medicine that the single trial decided on by the commission would be a "circus competition." Vallery-Radot states that during this period Pasteur was ap-

[1] Vallery-Radot, *ibid.*, p. 121.
[2] Garrison, *ibid.*, p. 620.
[3] Osler's Introduction to Vallery-Radot's *Life of Pasteur*, p. vii.
[4] Garrison, *ibid.*, p. 503.
[5] Vallery-Radot, *ibid.*, p. 83.

proved or blamed as a defender of a religious cause.[1] Some of this opposition was based on the desire for greater proof. Pasteur's dispute with Pouchet was obscured by the fact that Pouchet's hay infusion was much more difficult to sterilize than the yeast infusion employed by Pasteur.[2] Criticism of Pasteur's experiments on spontaneous generation by Dr. Charlton Bastian of London resulted in great opposition to all of Pasteur's later work, and opposition to Lister whose work was based on that of Pasteur.[3]

The belief in the spontaneity of disease as opposed to the germ theory of Pasteur, persisted among medical men for many years after Pasteur's experiments of 1862-66. Vallery-Radot states, " The theory of germs, the doctrine of virus ferments, all this was considered as a complete reversal of acquired notions, a heresy which had to be suppressed ".[4] Pasteur's treatment of rabies in 1870 was opposed by some because they still believed in the spontaneous origin of the disease.[5]

LeFort as late as 1878 believed that originally, before the propagation of the contagium germ, a purulent infection was spontaneously produced and developed.[6] The slowness of the diffusion of the germ theory may be ascribed to its novelty, to the opposition of authorities who augmented the " power of tradition ", and also to the fact that Pasteur's experiments were not entirely conclusive.

Pasteur's conclusions on anthrax met with some opposition also because of their novelty and because his " vaccine virus "

[1] Vallery-Radot, ibid., pp. 106-111.
[2] Garrison, ibid., p. 620.
[3] Vallery-Radot, ibid., pp. 252-6; Wrench, Life of Lister, p. 247; see later discussion of Lister.
[4] Vallery-Radot, ibid., p. 228.
[5] Vallery-Radot, ibid., p. 409.
[6] Vallery-Radot, ibid., p. 409.

for anthrax was by no means perfect. Davaine's announcement that he had isolated the anthrax germ had not been received without doubt and hesitation. Two research workers, Jaillard and Deplat were unsuccessful at arriving at the same result by experiment, and consequently sought to refute his conclusions. Paul Bert also opposed his view and supported Jaillard and Deplat.[1] The disbelief shown when Pasteur produced the vaccine against anthrax is indicated by a letter from Bouley after Pasteur's successful control experiment at a demonstration that had been arranged to discredit him. Bouley wrote,

The result is of special importance in a country side whose incredulity was being maintained in spite of all the demonstrations made. It seems that doctors especially were refractory. They said it was too good to be true and counted on the strength of the natural charbon to find your method in default.[2]

Koch and others contested the value of Pasteur's "vaccine virus" for anthrax because of their valid criticism of his method of preparing the vaccine.[3]

The opposition to Pasteur's conclusions on the diseases of the silk worm had its origin in ignorance, and vested interests which exploited this ignorance. The complicated proofs of Pasteur were incomprehensible to the simple seed growers who had to accept them on faith until they had tried the method of raising seeds themselves. All the precautions insisted upon seemed absurd to them. As stated previously, the fact that Pasteur was a chemist and not a sericulturist prejudiced them against his opinions. But the prime cause

[1] George Fleming, *Pasteur and His Work*, London, 1886, p. 34.

[2] In this experiment the sixteen sheep not inoculated previously with anthrax virus died and the vaccinated remained immune. See Vallery-Radot, *ibid.*, p. 328; DeKruif, *ibid.*, p. 159; L. Descour, *Pasteur and His Work*, pp. 192-4; S. J. Holmes, *Louis Pasteur*, pp. 174-8.

[3] Fleming, *ibid.*, p. 54.

for the hesitancy on the part of the silk-worm cultivators was the slanderous campaign of the seed merchants whose industry was gravely jeopardized by Pasteur's discovery. They spread malicious, fictitious reports of failures and created an antagonistic attitude toward the innovation. The character of the rumors which were circulated is indicated by a letter of M. Laurent to Madame Pasteur, "It is being reported here" (Lyons) "that the failure of Pasteur's process has excited the population of your neighborhood so much that he has had to flee from Alais, pursued by infuriated inhabitants throwing stones after him". The effect of this propaganda of the seed merchants defending their vested interests persisted for many years, and influenced the attitude of many to his other discoveries.[1]

The idea of partial heat sterilization or "pasteurization" was sceptically received. Those most concerned with the preservation of wine were at first incredulous as to the heating process not damaging its taste, color or limpidness. A large tasting commission appointed by the wholesale wine merchants of Paris could not agree as to the superiority of the heated or unheated wines at the first meeting, because of preconceptions, when they knew which wine they were drinking. At the second meeting, when they were not told which was the heated and which the unheated wine, they acknowledged that the difference between the two was imperceptible.[2]

All the devices of social pressure were employed against Pasteur. Attacks on his personality and the fact that he was a chemist, mentioned above,[3] indifference, and priority disputes[4] all were used to discourage the innovator and to detract from the value of his innovations.

[1] Vallery-Radot, *ibid.*, p. 156. See also *ibid.*, pp. 140, 121, 169-70, 207.
[2] Fleming, *ibid.*, p. 20.
[3] See the opposition of M. Peter, Vallery-Radot, *ibid.*, p. 365.
[4] E. g., Vallery-Radot, *ibid.*, p. 374.

OPPOSITION TO PASTEUR

Perhaps the greatest cause of opposition to Pasteur among the laity, was due to the vilefications of the anti-vivisectionists and the anti-vaccinationists. Pasteur received letters full of threats, insults and maledictions delivering him to eternal torments, because he used hens, guinea pigs, dogs and sheep in his laboratory experiments.[1] He was portrayed in the prodigious literature of the anti-vivisectionists as the "murderer of innocent animals", a "vile, murderous, rascally fiend", and his name came to be identified with cruelty.[2] A typical diatribe written in 1911 ends with the plea:

Extinguish Jennerism and Pasteurism and relieve the national and local treasuries of the burden of the parasites now foisted upon them by the Jennerian and Pasteurian cults—prohibit

[1] Vallery-Radot, *ibid.*, p. 334 *et seq.*

[2] The agitation against animal experimentation received its impetus in England in 1871, when J. Burdon Sanderson's *Handbook for the Physiological Laboratory* fell in the hands of people who, ignorant of vivisection, believed that no anaesthetics were used and that the medical student merely repeated experiments on animals for cruel pleasure. The movement reached such strength that in 1876 it produced the passage of a bill in England prohibiting vivisection. Since that time there has been constant agitation against vivisection in all countries of the world, several states in the United States having anti-vivisection laws, and in others the scientists must yearly fight against such laws. The proponents of the bills are, for the most part ignorant of the part animal experimentation has played in the knowledge and control of human and animal diseases; they look with horror upon the "needless torture" of animals and are encouraged in so doing by the literature of the anti-vivisection societies, illustrated by gruesome pictures denying the use of anaesthetics in the experiments. Psychologically, the emotion created is based on the principle of identification as in the case of dissection. See the anti-vivisection literature; also among the innumerable pamphlets on the subject, W. B. Cannon, *Anti-vivisection Legislation: Its History, Aims and Menace*; Cannon, *Some Characteristics of Anti-vivisection Literature*, 1911; F. A. Tondorf, *The Vindication of Vivisection*, 1923; W. Keen, *The Influence of Anti-vivisection on Character*, 1912; *Journal American Medical Association*, vol. 77, p. 792; vol. 79, p. 1448; vol. 84, p. 526.

the cruelties to children, to adults and to our humble animal brethren and friends which Jenner, Pasteur and their ignorant and dishonest followers daily commit.[1]

The anti-vaccinationists began to attack Pasteur when his experiments with anthrax in 1881 showed the validity of the principle of preventive inoculation. The English and American anti-vaccination movements were at their height at that time and these experiments were damaging to their cause. For this reason, they sought to discredit Pasteur and all his discoveries in an abusive campaign. The two following excerpts from the *Vaccination Inquirer* are illustrative:

There are no limits to credulity, any craze is possible; but audacity may be too audacious. Miraculous claims advanced in Pasteur's name have already passed into the category of illusions. We have not forgotten the abortive insurance company to make good the losses of stock under M. Pasteur's inoculation. There is evidently an active financial spirit associated with that savant and if only a furore can be excited over the cure of rabies by inoculation, the project of the Mansion House subscription will be revived. . . . Much of the praise lavished on Pasteur is inspired by the hope that he will yet redeem vaccination from the discredit that is gathering around it.[2] We renew our conviction that either M. Pasteur does not know what constitutes valid evidence or that he is deliberately practicing on public credulity for the sake of gain. His parade of cases of hydrophobia taken as cured, when he must know that the majority had nothing of hydrophobia about them, leaves him under the most odious imputation.[3]

The attacks of the anti-vivisectionists and the anti-vaccina-

[1] Montague R. Leverson, *Pasteur the Plagiarist*, p. 16; see also J. J. Garth Wilkinson, *Pasteur and Jenner, An Example and a Warning*.

[2] *Vaccination Inquirer*, vol. vii, p. 155.

[3] *Ibid.*, vol. viii, p. 114. See also The London Society for the Abolition of Compulsory Vaccination, Annual Meeting, 1886, p. 42 *et seq.*

tionists, given tremendous publicity, influenced masses of people to view Pasteur and his work with distrust and suspicion.

In summarizing the causes of the opposition to Pasteur, the factors provoking the resistance of the medical profession must again be distinguished from those determining the resistance of the masses. In the opposition of the former, may be distinguished the psychological factors, first, the tendency to suffuse an habitual mode of activity with an "emotional tone"; second, the persistence of habit reactions due to the difficulty of reconditioning behavior patterns; and third, the use of social pressure to exact conformity. The cultural factors were first, the conflict between Pasteur's theories and other medical theories supported by authorities of equal merit; second, the power of established authority; third, the rivalry between phases of culture in the form of the antagonism between medical men and research chemists; and fourth, ignorance as to the meaning and implications of the germ theory. The personality factor entered prominently in this instance.

In the opposition to Pasteur's seed innovations, which affected the attitude of many people toward his medical discoveries, can be discerned the psychological factors, first, of attaching an "emotional tone" to habitual activity, and second, the difficulty of reconditioning habitual behavior patterns. Most prominent, however, was the economic vested interests of the seed merchants who through propaganda, played upon the ignorance of the seed growers. The conflict between Pasteur and the anti-vaccinationists and anti-vivisectionists led these groups to exploit the ignorance of the masses to develop antagonism against Pasteur's work.

CHAPTER IX

OPPOSITION TO THE DOCTRINE OF ANTISEPSIS

THE opposition to the introduction of Lister's method of antiseptic surgery was intense. Cheyne portrays the conflict between the supporters of Lister and others in Edinburgh where

The non-Listerians looked on the others as crazy believers in vain things like germs, rash to a degree, blinded by their enthusiasm, placing their patients in the greatest danger by the outrageous treatment they proposed, and as they said that their wounds did not suppurate while those of the other side did, liars of the first water.[1]

London surgeons were bitterly antagonistic. Dr. Just Lucas Championniere, the most persistent advocate of Lister's method in France wrote, " . . . I was subject to a sort of persecution on the part of those whose scientific repose I was violently upsetting ".[2] Von Nussbaum in Germany stated in 1887,

Ten years ago, many distinguished surgeons called Lister's treatment humbug and considered it an unpardonable attack on surgical freedom to assert that no surgeon has a right to be ignorant of the antiseptic treatment. In 1880, I said in a clinical lecture that in medico-legal cases a surgeon could be called to account if he completely ignored antiseptics and lost a patient from pyaemia. For this I was reproached in a most violent manner both verbally and in print. A distinguished medical

[1] W. Cheyne, *Lister and His Achievement*, p. 25.
[2] R. Godlee, *Lord Lister*, 1917, p. 353.

jurist wrote a letter about me in which he called me a fanatic and said that no medical jurist alive would reproach a practical surgeon who acted faithfully according to the teaching of the text books, recommended at the University, because a practical surgeon could neither buy all new books, nor ought he to allow his principles to be shaken by every new discovery.[1]

In 1875, Theodore Billroth of Vienna wrote to Volkmann, " If you were not so energetic a supporter of this (the antiseptic) method, I should say that the whole thing was a swindle ".[2] Stephen Smith comments that when he introduced Lister's method into the wards of the Bellevue Hospital, many of his colleagues were disgusted and refused even to visit the wards when the patients were under treatment.[3]

The most evident cause of the slowness of the acceptance of Lister's innovation of antisepsis was the novelty of the germ theory upon which his work was based. At the meeting of the British Medical Association at Leeds, in 1869, Mr. Nunneley, who delivered the address on surgery, articulated this opposition.

The theory and reasoning by which the antiseptic treatment of wounds is supported, appear to overlook facts open to all the world, to disregard observations familiar to every person through all ages from the earliest period to the present day. . . . We may probably with safety deny the existence of germs in the number and universality maintained by Pasteur and Lister.[4]

In 1870, Dr. James Morton, formerly a surgeon to the

[1] Godlee, *ibid.*, p. 340.

[2] Godlee, *ibid.*, p. 349.

[3] Reminiscences of Two Epochs—Anesthesia and Asepsis, *Johns Hopkins Hospital Bulletin*, vol. xxx, p. 277 *et seq.*

[4] G. T. Wrench, *Lord Lister*, 1914, London, p. 193; R. Godlee, *ibid.*, p. 311.

Glasgow Infirmary, wrote a letter to the *Lancet* concerning Lister's method, in which he said that " Pasteur's theory in regard to the existence of certain spores or germs in the air " had not been satisfactorily proven.[1] Robert Lawson Tait, the famous English ovariotomist declined to see any relation between bacteria and disease.[2] In France, M. Le Fort maintained : " That theory (the germ theory) in its applications to clinical surgery, is absolutely inacceptable. . . . I believe in the interiority of the principle of purulent infection in certain patients; that is why I oppose the extension to surgery of the germ theory which proclaims constant *exteriority* of that principle ".[3] Theodore Billroth, in Vienna, who followed Liebig in denying that micro-organisms caused decomposition wrote, in 1874, " That which of late years is often lovingly called the antiseptic treatment, is in my opinion only a potential ' Antiplegmonous ' or as it used to be commonly called ' Antiplogistic ' treatment of wounds ".[4] Robert Weir in 1878 asserted that the most weighty objection to Lister's method in America was the positiveness of the enunciation of the germ theory in explanation of the process of decomposition in the secretions of a wound.[5]

Not understanding the fundamental theory back of Lister's practice, many men who were willing to give the new method a trial failed to secure the same results as Lister. They regarded his treatment a " mere method of dressing " or laid stress on the use of carbolic acid, disregarding the minutiae in the practice upon whic hits success depended. Among these was James Paget, who made public his

[1] Godlee, *ibid.*, pp. 250-1.
[2] Garrison, *ibid.*, p. 649.
[3] Vallery-Radot, *ibid.*, p. 270 *et seq.*
[4] Godlee, *ibid.*, p. 348.
[5] Robert E. Weir, *On the Antiseptic Treatment of Wounds*, New York, 1878, *passim.*

failures and thus retarded the acceptance of the new method.[1] These repeated failures provoked an editorial in the *Lancet* which concluded with the statement,

Happily it is no part of the clinical surgeon to bolster up theories whether they be good or bad, or to make facts rigidly to conform to them. The germ theory may be perfectly well founded but nine out of ten surgeons do not much care whether it is or not, so long as they cure their cases and reduce their mortality to the lowest possible degree.[2]

The failures caused earlier apathy in England to pass into opposition and to mention antiseptic surgery was to cause irritation, or at least to occasion a scoff or a sneer, as is evidenced in the debate at the Clinical Society of London in 1875.[3] For the same reason by 1875, the earlier enthusiasm in Germany had cooled so that in some places actual opposition set in. In Holland, Belgium, South Germany and Vienna the treatment had been tried and given up. Surgeons were content to apply carbolic acid dressings to the wounds and suppurating surfaces and to look upon Lister's publications with distrust.[4]

The opposition to Lister was strengthened by the rejection of the method by the famous surgeon, James Simpson. Simpson's opposition was due to the fact that he looked upon the antiseptic treatment as a rival to an invention of his own, known as "acupressure" simply because they both aimed at procuring healing without suppuration. Simpson was mortified that although brilliant results were reported from Aberdeen, his method was not used in Edinburgh or Glasgow. He sent an anonymous letter to the *Edinburgh Daily Review* on September 23, 1867, signed "Chirurgious", stating that

[1] C. Dukes. *Lord Lister*, London, 1924, p. 120 *et seq.*
[2] *Lancet*, 1875, vol. ii, p. 597.
[3] Godlee, *ibid.*, p. 320.
[4] Godlee, *ibid.*, p. 343.

Lister had been antedated by Lemaire and others in the use of carbolic acid. The letter was circulated by Simpson and commented on in the *Lancet*, where it was insinuated that Lister had merely reproduced a continental practice. Lister, in replying, acknowledged the priority of Lemaire whose work he had not known previously, and then showed that his work implied more than the mere use of carbolic acid. Simpson answered in a bitter attack under the title of "Carbolic Acid and its Compounds in Surgery", in which he accused Lister of the most culpable ignorance of medical literature and negated the value of the antiseptic treatment compared with the results obtained by "acupressure", asking why Lister and other surgeons persisted in rejecting a practice which had given such excellent results. Simpson's opposition to Lister, provoked by his vested interest in "acupressure", was further aggravated by his persistent antagonism to John Symes, Lister's chief and father-in-law.[1] The authority of Simpson afforded many conservative surgeons the excuse they sought to make it unnecessary for them to change their established habits.

There were other rival systems that claimed excellent results supported by highly competent authorities. Humphry of Cambridge advocated the "open method"; Spence used warm water and iodine; Callender trusted to cleanliness alone.[2] Gamgee of Birmingham testified as to Lister's good results but said that Lister had unwisely ignored "the marvelous efficacy of two such remedial principles as compression and suspension and does not at the same time weigh the relative advantages of moist and dry, frequent and rare dressings".[3] Others still believed in "laudable pus".[4] In

---

[1] Wrench, *ibid.*, pp. 141-2, 150, 177 *et seq.*; Godlee, *ibid.*, p. 199 *et seq.*; Dukes, *ibid.*, p. 115 *et seq.*

[2] Godlee, *ibid.*, p. 320 *et seq.*; Cheney, *ibid.*, p. 41.

[3] Wrench, *ibid.*, p. 249 *et seq.*

[4] Drinkwater, *Fifty Years of Medical Progress*, Preface; Stephen Smith, *op. cit.*, p. 276.

France, the *pansement ouate* of Alphonse Guerin was set up in opposition to Lister's treatment and held its own until 1880.[1] Dr. Kronlein in Germany defended by statistical data an " open treatment ", as being superior to the antiseptic method. Surgeons were therefore naturally hesitant in accepting the antiseptic method, especially since doubt had been cast upon its efficacy and because it further involved effort to perform the minute precautions demanded. These precautions they dismissed with ridicule.[2]

Lister's erroneous insistence on the use of the antiseptic spray machine whose purpose it was to create an antiseptic atmosphere surrounding the wound, made some of the opposition to his method well grounded. The spray gave a great sense of security to those who believed that the germs of the air infected the wound, but it made the operation an unnecessary ordeal. When the vapor was too coarse, the hands of the operator were made numb and white by the carbolic acid lotion. The carbonised steam passed into the lungs whenever the spray was used and when operations were performed in a room illuminated by gas or lamps, the gas set free irritated the operator. Many surgeons upon whom the effect of carbolic acid was deleterious could not use the spray. It was undoubtedly the cause also of many cases among the patients of carbolic acid poisoning following operations.

Doubts were cast from time to time as to the utility of the spray even by some of Lister's loyal followers. The opposition culminated in a paper by Bruns of Tübingen in 1880, entitled *Fort Mit Dem Spray,* in which he suggested a return to irrigation used previous to 1871 by Lister. Many surgeons then abandoned its use; but Lister, although he spoke hesitatingly about it at the International Medical Con-

[1] Godlee, *ibid.*, p. 352.
[2] L. Descour, *Pasteur and his Work*, 1922, p. 142; Valley-Radot, *ibid.*, p. 239.

gress in 1881, persisted in employing it until 1887. He finally relinquished it because Keith and other ovariotomists who did not use the spray, were as effective as those who did, because Metchnicoff's discovery of phagocytosis showed that invading microorganisms were devoured by phagocytes, and because the accumulating weight of evidence showed that pathogenic organisms were not very plentiful in the air and that the source of wound infection was the patient's skin, the surgeon's hands, unsterilised sponges and instruments and particles of dirt of all kinds. After years of persistent advocacy, even after others had seen the uselessness of the spray, Lister said in 1890, at the International Medical Congress in Berlin, " I feel ashamed that I should ever have recommended it (the spray) for the purpose of destroying the microbes of the air." The controversy about the spray was a tremendous factor in delaying the diffusion of Lister's theory of germ infection.[1] All who wished to discredit Lister referred to his position on the spray machine.[2]

Attacks upon the antiseptic method also came from those who attributed the decline in hospital diseases and mortality to improvement in hospital hygiene, to isolation, ventilation and avoidance of overcrowding, and to the improvement of nursing. Such was the opinion of a considerable proportion of the senior members of the staffs of London and provincial hospitals who were concerned with these problems. It was expressed at the meeting of the British Medical Association at Cork in 1879 by Wm. Savory, who demanded statistics to prove the value of antiseptics and insinuated that Lister was suppressing statistics because he had none that he was not ashamed to produce. It is but natural that this scepti-

---

[1] Godlee, *ibid.*, p. 284 *et seq.*; Dukes, *ibid.*, pp. 144-5.

[2] *E. g.*, in 1914 the *Vaccination Inquirer* referred to the "lunatic Listerism which tried to kill imaginary germs by directing carbolic acid spray on to the wounds on the operating table," vol. xxxvi, p. 276.

cism and criticism of antisepsis should have been provoked because of the revolutionary changes in hospital technique independent of the antiseptic method, because of the many failures of those who had tried the process, because of the absence of convincing statistics and because of the powerful influence of James Simpson.[1]

Some of the opposition to Lister was provoked by a desire to defend institutions and individuals from his criticism. When Lister left Glasgow in 1870, he wrote a paper "On the Effects of the Antiseptic System of Treatment upon the Salubrity of a Surgical Hospital". In it he described the vicious conditions existing in the hospital while he was securing excellent results by the use of the antiseptic method. He stated that his own wards had been "converted from some of the most unhealthy in the Kingdom into models of healthiness". This nettled the directors who were concerned with the reputation of their hospital and some of Lister's former colleagues who felt that he was trying to glorify himself at their expense.[2]

Similar irritable indignation was aroused by a report of an impromptu speech of Lister to his class at Edinburgh which appeared in the *London Times* of February 23, 1877, in which he said that "he considered the system of teaching in Surgery in Edinburgh much superior to that pursued in London". London surgeons made sharp comments on this report, assuming that the criticism had been directed against individuals. The *Lancet* fulminated editorially

. . . like a man who in the excitement of enthusiasm raves at the false creations of his heat oppressed brain, Mr. Lister fancied he saw his professional confreres in London only unsubstantial shades and showy shams. . . . In many quarters, Mr. Lister has

---
[1] Godlee, *ibid.*, p. 321 *et seq.*
[2] Godlee, *ibid.*, pp. 246-251; Dukes, *ibid.*, p. 129.

acquired the reputation of a thoughtful, painstaking surgeon and has done some service to practical surgery by insisting on the importance of cleanliness in the treatment of wounds, although this has been done by the glorification of an idea which is neither original nor universally accepted, but even these circumstances do not warrant him in arrogating to himself the right to sit in judgment on his fellows and publicly denounce as imposters those who have the misfortune to differ from him.[1]

This controversy accounts for the apathy and indifference to Lister's teaching when he first came to London. The examiners were Lister's antagonists and the students desirous of passing the examinations avoided Lister's courses.[2]

The cost of carbolic acid dressings compared to water dressings retarded the introduction of the antiseptic method. The Board of the Edinburgh Infirmary complained about the expense involved.[3] In Munich, von Nussbaum was obliged to counter the argument of excessive cost.[4] Lister pointed out that von Bardeleben would have attained better results had he not, on the score of economy, substituted unprepared gauze soaked in a solution of carbolic acid instead of using antiseptic gauze.[5]

We find involved in opposition to Lister the hesitancy of accepting an innovation that was only one of the many innovations attempting to meet a certain need, the efficacy of which was disputed by authorities, some of whom are reported to have given the method a trial, the practice of which involved a change of habits, discomfort and additional effort, and which was based on a theory of disease which was still a matter of controversy. The devices of ridicule and dis-

[1] *Lancet*, 1877, vol. i, p. 361; Godlee, *ibid.*, p. 397 *et seq.*
[2] Cheyne, *op. cit.*, p. 34; Godlee, *op. cit.*, p. 417; Duke, *op. cit.*, p. 155.
[3] Wrench, *ibid.*, p. 251.
[4] Wrench, *ibid.*, p. 256.
[5] Godlee, *ibid.*, p. 342.

paragement by priority controversies, the emphasis on the questionable phases of Lister's method such as the use of the spray, the vested interests of those whose theories were conflicting with Lister's, the acrimony of those whose reputations were at stake due to failure to apply the method, intensified and protracted the antagonism to antisepsis as a surgical principle. The psychological factors that can be discerned, therefore, are first, the tendency to suffuse a habitual mode of activity with an "emotional tone" or psychological vested interest; second, fear reaction in the presence of the unknown; third, the persistence of habit reactions due to the difficulty of reconditioning behavior patterns; fourth, the avoidance of the unpleasant; fifth, the mechanism of rationalization, and sixth, the use of social pressure to exact conformity. The cultural factors were first, the power of authority; second, vested interests; third, ignorance; fourth, the role of money; and fifth, the conflict with other medical theories. Personality conflicts also contributed to the resistance to the innovation.

CHAPTER X

Opposition to Asepsis

WHEN asepsis was introduced by von Bergmann and formulated and developed by Simmelbusch in 1892, as a substitute for antisepsis, it was the proponents of Lister's method rather than the more conservative surgeons who opposed it. They had attached such vehement emotional tone to their practice, they had such a psychological vested interest in it, that they resented any improvement upon it and developed rationalizations to justify its retention.

Lister himself, though not as violent an opponent as some of his followers, expressed himself against asepsis, " . . . it has grieved me to learn that many surgeons have been led to substitute needlessly protracted and complicated measures for means so simple and efficient (as the antiseptic) ".[1] Hector Cameron, Lister's friend, maintained in 1907 that Lister deplored the complications which he knew from his experience to be wholly superfluous. He adds his own complaint that because of the architectural and mechanical arrangements, the amount of skilled assistance required, the use of gloves, masks and other accessories, surgery was to be confined to a splendidly equipped hospital eliminating ordinary surgical practice.[2] Dr. Lucas Champonniere, in France, denounced asepsis in 1902,

This surgery is nothing more than laboratory work. . . . Never before have the architects been more indispensable. The least defect in the condition of an operating room manifests itself by disasters. If the surgeon does not surround himself with im-

---

[1] J. B. Lister, *Collected Papers*, Oxford, 1908, vol. ii, p. 370.
[2] Wrench, *ibid.*, p. 326.

OPPOSITION TO ASEPSIS

practicable precautions—masks, gloves, etc.,—the safety of the patient is imperilled. The old surgical world protested against the easy going and regular precautions which Lister took. Modern surgeons, instead of moderating these precautions which might be moderated, introduce new and incredible precautions incompatible with regular practice. And yet have they altered the results of surgery? Certainly they have caused it to lose its safety.[1]

The objections of the "Listerians" to asepsis are most vehemently and querulously expressed by Wrench:

Lister did not use the nailbrush, which he regarded as superfluous. He did not scrub his hands for so many minutes by the watch nor soak them in several lotions. He did not use boiled gloves, boiled robes, boiled cap, boiled mask or boiled muzzle. He remained an ordinary human being to the eye of the spectator. He was not attired like a mummer at a carnival. He never adopted all these 'improvements' because he had faith in his own observations of the power that carbolic acid possessed of rendering and keeping organic matter aseptic.[2] The avoidance of septic disaster, quite apart from surgical skill, instead of being represented as a reward of faithful adherence to Listerism, is shown to the student to be dependent—and even then it is not assured—upon an enormous and expensive equipment of various forms of sterilizers, autoclaves, mosaic floors, tiled walls, sterilized water, air filterers, highly trained assistants, boiled robes boiling a short time to rag, boiled gloves soon becoming rotten, boiled instruments soon becoming blunt, architectural rotundities and mechanical specialties, which can only be enjoyed at hospitals by the charity of the public and at nursing homes by the largeness of the fees, by quite a limited number of surgeons. The certain benefits of Lister which could have been spread through the land in cottage as well as in palace, have been converted into a ring and a fetish. The student walking the hospital instead of being

[1] Wrench, *ibid.*, p. 326 *et seq.*
[2] Wrench, *ibid.*, p. 324.

taught the beautiful simplicity and mastery of Lister, is like an acolyte instructed in mysteries; but should he not join the peculiar priesthood, he eventually finds himself turned out upon the world, dubious and incompetent, because he has not at his beck and call the elaborate paraphernalia of a palatial modern hospital. Surgery, in a word, has been not only rendered unsafe but it has been made an expensive monopoly of the surgeons who get attached to the public hospitals. Not only does the student and future practitioner suffer gravely from this rapid departure from the simplicity of Lister, but the ever-increasing cost to the public is enormous. "The need of asepsis" says a writer upon the London Hospital and its construction and outfit which he admires, "has led to an enormous expenditure which becomes a fixed and permanent expenditure." [1]

Even Godlee, though admitting the superior value of the modern aseptic methods, disparages them by pointing out that the idea was not new.[2]

The antiseptic-aseptic controversy affords an excellent illustrative example of an innovation affording a transition stage to a more efficacious method, only to retard the reception of a new development, by involving all the typical, psychological, cultural and mechanical factors at the basis of opposition to change.

[1] Wrench, *ibid.*, p. 331 *et seq.*
[2] Godlee, *ibid.*, p. 452 *et seq.*

CHAPTER XI

Summary

To avoid oversimplification and to portray the subtler shades of the controversies relating to resistance to new methods and ideas in the history of medicine, the causes of opposition to specific innovations have been analysed critically. It has been observed that in each instance, the immediate setting of the innovation, and the nature of the innovation itself, determine the forces that will be brought into play against it, preventing its diffusion. It may be of some value, however, to enumerate the number of times each of the factors analysed in chapter one, has been found to be present in the specific instances studied.

The psychological factors, the tendency to suffuse an habitual mode of activity with an "emotional tone" that gives it an exaggerated value, and the persistence of habit reactions due to the difficulty of reconditioning behavior patterns, are found in all of the eight examples studied. Social pressure is the next prominent psychological factor, involved as it is in all instances but that of percussion. It is difficult to determine with certainty when rationalizations are employed, but they appear in an obvious manner in the opposition to dissection and vaccination, both among physicians and laymen, and in the resistance to antisepsis and asepsis. In these four instances, fear and the avoidance of pain and the unpleasant are also found.

That ignorance, based on inability to weigh the relative merits of conflicting theories, results in the investing of authority with great power, with subsequent retarding of innovations is substantiated by all the specific instances studied. Economic vested interests were involved in the opposition to dissection, vaccination, Pasteur, antisepsis and asepsis. Conflicts with other phases of culture which served to arouse mass opposition to medical innovations are illustrated in the antagonism to dissection, to Pasteur and to vaccination.

The mechanical difficulties of diffusing knowledge played a large role in delaying the recognition of Auenbrugger's theory of percussion, and also has been one of the factors which has prolonged the mass opposition to vaccination. Dissection and vaccination, dependent as they have been on legislation, have been retarded by the delays attendant on legislative activity. Asepsis could not be practised until adequate hospital facilities were provided, which occasioned a mechanical delay even after the principle was accepted.

Personality conflicts were important in retarding the acceptance of vaccination, Semmelweis's theory of the nature of puerperal fever, the discoveries of Pasteur, and to a lesser degree, the quarrel between Simpson and John Symes affected the opposition to the antiseptic method.

No inference is made that the factors summarized above will be found in a like proportion in the general field of medical conservatism or in other fields when opposition to innovations occurs. Furthermore, the limitations of the summary are obvious because each factor listed is not of the same intensity in any of the controversies, and although certain factors may be classified under the same heading, they function in a distinctly different manner in the various instances considered. The summary, therefore, serves only to sum up in a very general way, the factors involved in the examples studied in detail, as a supplement to the formulation of the hypotheses derived from the data, given in chapter one.

PART II
THE NATURE OF MEDICAL PROGRESS

CHAPTER I

BIOGRAPHY IN MEDICAL HISTORY

MEDICAL history has until recently been for the most part, a study of biographies. Individuals who have contributed to the development of medicine are lauded with panegyrics, and, isolated from their social and scientific background, are given exaggerated importance as initiators of new diagnostic methods, or discoverers of long-sought-after causal relations or cures. The popular view of the individual's place in the history of medicine is indicated by Jacobi's statement: " . . . in arts and sciences, it is individual brains and exertions that have created sudden wonders which caused permanent changes in knowledge and convictions and resulted in practical reforms and revolutions,"[1] and Longcope's comment

Throughout the development of medicine it is apparent that real progress, lasting progress, has come only from individual effort expended in scientific investigation, whether this be purely inductive as was the method of Hippocrates or experimental as was the method of Harvey or Pasteur. It is upon the individual working silently for years, unhampered free of thought, usually unappreciated that we must depend for the idea, the jewel upon which the wheel will turn.[2]

Osler quotes with approval Disraeli's statement, " A great nation is a nation which produces great men " and remarks

[1] Victor Robinson, *Pathfinders in Medicine*, p. 7.
[2] Longcope, " Milestones in Medicine," *Educational Review*, 1916, vol. 52, p. 348.

that Pasteur looked upon the cult of great men as an important principle in national education as is indicated by his dicta to the students of the University of Edinburgh—" Worship great men." [1]

The works of Karl Sudhoff in Germany and Charles Singer in England on ancient and medieval medicine indicate clearly that movements and traditions in medicine can be studied irrespective of individuals. Singer's method is exemplified by his comment in a discussion of a medical commentary of the first half of the twelfth century.

The history of medicine consists essentially of a successive series of intellectual movements proceeding from different centers and each engulfing its predecessor. Our manuscript exhibits the Anglo-Saxon medicine in the actual process of absorption by the doctrines of Salerno. In another century, Salerno became lost in the intellectual invasion that spread from Cordova to Bagdad. The Arabian system again gave place to the Greek medicine that was received with the rise of Humanism, until Renaissance science was in its turn lost in that great flood of ideas introduced by the Experimental Method.[2]

Garrison's *History of Medicine,* great as is its value, is primarily and even effusively biographical. That the author is alertly conscious of the problem is shown by his deference to the criticism of Welch that he had not written a history of medicine as an inductive science and his endorsement of Singer's statement that " The history of medicine is a history of ideas and biography is only of value insofar as it bears on ideas." [3]

In analyzing the causative factors in any invention or discovery in medicine, in an attempt to determine the extent

---
[1] Introduction to Vallery-Radot, *Life of Pasteur*, p. xv.
[2] *Bulletin Medical History,* Chicago, vol. ii, no. 1, p. 96.
[3] F. H. Garrison, *History of Medicine,* 2nd ed., pp. 7-8.

of the individual's contribution, the questions will be considered as to what degree the elements which enter into the discovery are dependent upon prior work in the field of medicine and in how far developments in fields independent of medicine affect the discovery. An attempt will be made to ascertain whether the discovery would have been made irrespective of the individual who is now heralded as the discoverer; in other words, whether it was inevitable or dependent upon the work of any particular genius.

CHAPTER II

The Dependence of a Discovery upon the Existing Knowledge

MEDICAL discoveries and inventions whether they be in the descriptive field of anatomy, in the diagnosis of causal relations between pathogenic microorganisms and a specific disease, in the realm of immunology, or in surgery and therapeutics, have not been made suddenly, but have been preceded by a multitude of preliminary and progressive steps which in turn had their antecedents. This principle applies without exception, even to those medical discoveries and practices which are popularly considered as the result of the epoch-making work of some individual. A few such instances will be analyzed.

The common opinion that Vesalius sprang like Minerva from the head of Jove and broke the record of previous ages by dissecting the human body for the first time does not bear critical examination.[1] It was the combination of

[1] Frederick II (1194-1250) ordained as early as 1231 that a public dissection of the human body be held at least once in five years at Salerno. The beginning of human dissection in anatomical study at Bologna was in the decade between 1266 and 1275. The chronicle of the Franciscan, Salimbene of Parma, written in 1288 gives the first frank reference to post-mortem examination in a statement that a physician of Cremona opened a corpse to see if he could find the cause of the pestilence that raged in Italy in 1286. The first formal account of a definite post-mortem examination was in 1302, when two physicians and three surgeons with Bartholmo de Variganana at their head reported on a certain Azzolino who died at Bologna under suspicious circumstances. Singer found in the Bodleian Library an illustration of Norman or Anglo-Norman workmanship, which can be dated about 1300, showing a surgeon opening a body and extracting the organs in the presence of a physician

humanist intellectual activity and the new naturalist art that
and a monk. The pictures used by Henri de Mondeville who after
studying at Bologna gave lectures in anatomy at Montpellier indicate
the manner of human dissection at that time. Mondino systematically
dissected the human body in public at Bologna 1300-1325.
Records of the practice of dissection in the 14th and 15th centuries are
numerous. Louis of Anjou in 1376 permitted the surgeons of Montpellier to take the body of an executed criminal annually for dissection.
Charles the Bad, King of Navarre, ratified this grant in 1377 as did
Charles VI in 1396 and Charles VIII in 1484 and 1496. The statutes of
Florence dated 1387 ordered the bodies of criminals to be delivered for
dissection. Venice decreed annual dissections in 1368 but they were not
performed. In 1404, Galeatus de Sancti Sophia came from Padua to
Venice to perform a public dissection which lasted a week. The next
public dissection in Venice was in 1416 and the dissection of a woman's
body was first permitted in 1452. When the University of Prague was
founded in 1348, executioners were enjoined to deliver the cadavers of
malefactors to the school of medicine. King John of Aragon in 1391,
directed that bodies of criminals be delivered to the University of Lerida.
At Bologna, dissection was recognized in the University statutes in 1405
and in 1442 it was decreed that one male and one female corpse should
be dissected annually. The same decree was enacted in Padua where a
male criminal had been dissected in 1429 and a female in the following
year, and also in Ferrara and Pisa. Public dissections were held at
Paris in 1478 and 1493 and in Tübingen in 1485. Vienna passed statutes
regulating dissection in 1497. Doubtless the number of dissections was
greater than these desultory records show.

Immediately preceding Vesalius, "the humanist anatomists": Johannes
Gunther (1487-1574), Sylvius (Jacques Dubois) of Paris (1478-1555)
and Charles Estienne (Stephanus) (-1564) were prominent as dissectors of the human body. The desire of the artists and the sculptors
to portray the human body realistically stimulated them to dissect the
human body for themselves. Verrocchio (1435-88), Andrea Mantegna
(died 1506), Lucia Signorelli (1444?-1524), Pollajuolo (1429-1498),
Donatello (1386-1466), Leonardo da Vinci (1452-1519), Albrecht Dürer
(1471-1528), Michelangelo (1475-1564) and Raphael (1483-1521) all used
the scalpel on the human body. See F. Baker, "The Two Sylviuses,"
Bulletin Johns Hopkins Hospital, vol. xx (1909), p. 329 *et seq.*; T.
Puschman, *The History of Medical Education*, pp. 246, 249-50; G. Fischer,
Chirurgie vor 100 Jahren, 1876, p. 94 *et seq.*; C. Singer, *Evolution of
Anatomy*; E. C. Streeter, "The Role of Certain Florentines in the History of Anatomy," *Bulletin Johns Hopkins Hospital*, vol. xxvii, p.
113 *et seq.*

brought forth Vesalius as a characteristic product of his age. As Singer writes:

> Until these two had come together there could be no Vesalius. When these two had come together, there had to be a Vesalius. . . . (He was) trebly equipped for his task; first by his own native genius for dissection developed with Sylvius at Paris and stimulated by the freedom of teaching at Padua; secondly, by the current attitude toward the human body exalted by contact with the Renaissance Art; thirdly, by an admirable education according to the standards of the time, directed along humanistic lines by Gunther, one of the ablest medical humanists of the day.[1]

There has even been an extended controversy as to whether Vesalius plagiarized from Leonardo da Vinci.[2]

Harvey's work also was a product of his time in the sense that it was the inevitable result of the humanist movement and the existing status of medical knowledge. There is no doubt of his dependence upon Aristotle whose work he knew and acknowledged.[3] Pulmonary circulation had been described by the martyred Michael Servetus, whose ideas were appropriated by Realdus Columbus (1559). Caesalpinus (1519-1603), who was the first to use the term *circulatio* in speaking of the movement of the blood, anticipated Harvey in holding that the blood returns from the general tissues to the heart by the veins alone. Fabricus ab Aquapendente (1537-1613), Harvey's teacher, had demonstrated in a complete manner the valves of the veins. Harvey's contribution

---

[1] C. Singer, *Evolution of Anatomy*, pp. 110, 114.

[2] The controversy opened by E. Jackscath (*Med. Bl.*, Wien, 1902, vol. xxv, pp. 770-772) and participated in by Forster, Hull, Roth, Sudhoff and others has been decided in the negative. See F. H. Garrison, "In Defence of Vesalius," *Bulletin of Society Medical History*, Chicago, vol. i, no. 4, pp. 47-65; A. Klebs, "Leonardo da Vinci and his Anatomical Studies," *ibid.*, p. 66-83.

[3] Raymond Crawfurd, "Forerunners of Harvey in Antiquity," *British Medical Journal*, 1919, vol. ii, pp. 551-556.

was the corroboration by the experimental method of the "clever guesses" of Caesalpinus and Servetus. His dependence upon the existing technic is further shown by the fact that his demonstration of circulation was incomplete because he could not see capillary anastomosis between arteries and veins, having no microscope.[1] That the experimental method was becoming established in Harvey's time is shown by the work of his contemporaries in physics and astronomy and by the *Novum Organum* of Francis Bacon, written at this time.[2]

Morgagni, credited with laying the foundation of modern pathological anatomy, acknowledged his independence on the previous post-mortems of Bonet and Benivieni, and Vesalius had also recognized the importance of diseased viscera in the dead body.[3] Wells and Blackall had established the correlation between dropsy and albuminous urine before Richard Bright made his celebrated synthesis.[4]

Vaccination was not a distinctive innovation on the part of Jenner. The immunity to small pox which cow pox affords was known widely in Great Britain and on the continent, its protective power had been discussed before medical societies and had been shown experimentally prior to Jenner. Vaccination, which was the logical outcome of variation or inoculation of small-pox virus, had been performed by Benjamin Jesty in England and Jensen and Plett in Germany.

[1] Robert Willis, *Works of William Harvey*, Preface; F. Baker, "History of Anatomy" in *Reference Book of the Medical Sciences* (Wood, 1923), vol. i, p. 331 *et seq.*; Arnold Chaplin, "Medicine in the Century before Harvey," *British Medical Journal*, 1922, vol. ii, pp. 707 *et seq.*; D. F. Harris, "Harvey versus Caesalpinus." Seventeenth International Congress of Medicine, Proceedings of Section on History of Medicine, London, 1913, vol. xxiii, p. 351.
[2] R. H. Moon, *The Relation of Medicine to Philosophy*, p. 144.
[3] F. H. Garrison, *History of Medicine*, 3rd ed., p. 363.
[4] Garrison, *ibid.*, p. 441.

To Jenner alone cannot even be ascribed the credit for convincing the world of the efficacy of the method, for without the work of Pearson and Woodville, his book would probably have received little attention.[1]

Pasteur's discovery of molecular dyssemmetry which led to his further work on the study of ferments and microörganisms would not have been possible without the prior work of Scheele, Gay-Lussac, Mitscherlich and Malus.[2] Latour and Schwann had discovered the organic nature of yeast and prepared the way for Pasteur's work on fermentation.[3] Redi, Spallanzani, Vallisneri and others had already propounded the doctrine, *omne vivum ex vivo*.[4] In his investigations on anthrax, Pasteur was preceded by Davaine who had discovered the bacillus and shown that the virulence of the disease was in proportion to the number of bacteria present; by Klebs, who indicated that the anthrax virus was not filterable and by Koch, who first cultivated pure cultures of anthrax bacilli, described their full life history and their relation to the disease.[5] Toussaint of Toulouse had preceded Pasteur in successfully inoculating with the anthrax virus, and Sanderson and Greenfield, in England, had discovered the method independently and simultaneously.[6] The diplococcus of pneumonia was isolated in 1880 by George Sternberg in the United States independently and prior to Pasteur.[7] Koch's famous " postulates " establishing the patho-

[1] Bernhard J. Stern, *Should We Be Vaccinated: A Survey of the Controversy in its Historical and Scientific Aspects*, New York, 1927, p. 4 *et seq.*

[2] Vallery-Radot, *Life of Pasteur*, p. 38 *et seq.*

[3] *Ibid.*, p. 80.

[4] *Ibid.*, p. 89 *et seq.*

[5] Garrison, *ibid.*, p. 621.

[6] Geo. Fleming, *Pasteur and His Work*, London, 1886, p. 52.

[7] Garrison, *ibid.*, p. 627.

genic character of a given microörganism, had already been developed by Henle and Klebs.[1] Semmelweis in Vienna, anticipated in many respects the work of Lister which was based on Pasteur.[2] The important discoveries of Loeffler, Gaffky, von Behring, Metchnikoff, Roux, Yersin, Kitasato and other immunologists, bacteriologists, and parisitologists, were and are dependent on an ever-accumulating knowledge based on the foundations established by Pasteur, Koch and the previous investigators.

The above facts do not tend to depreciate the contributions of the men under discussion nor to imply that they were negligible and unimportant. That years of patient and indefatigible research were involved is not overlooked or disparaged. It is acknowledged that there are variations in the importance of inventions and discoveries, that the accumulation of knowledge in medicine is not gradually continuous but is characterized by sudden spurts. Pending a particular discovery or one of a class, further progress, further discoveries in a given field are impossible. When the discovery is made, numerous developments follow immediately when investigators apply themselves to the field. This is well illustrated in modern medicine by the discoveries in the field of pathogenic microörganisms after the work of Pasteur and Koch.

The "key" discoveries, however, are in turn dependent upon antecedent discoveries which are indispensable. The preliminary discoveries, seemingly insignificant when evaluated pragmatically, often require as much or at times more persistent effort in research than the discovery which is considered important. The latter may involve only a very slight change in the formulation of a method or a minute variation of the knowledge already accumulated. Yet as a

[1] Garrison, *ibid.*, p. 623.
[2] J. W. Sinclair, *Semmelweis, His Life and Doctrine, passim.*

rule, the antecedent cultural base is minimized if not entirely overlooked in accounts of the important discovery.

A discovery in medicine is not only limited by the status of knowledge in medicine, but it is dependent upon the existing knowledge in other fields. An analysis of the field of experimental medicine will illustrate this fact vividly.

The extent of the dependence of experimental medicine upon the developments in other fields of knowledge shows how minute is the contribution of any particular individual compared to the vast accumulation of knowledge upon which his work is based. He uses metals, rubber, glass, asbestos, cement, lenses, motors, batteries, gas and innumerable other basic substances, a mere list of which, without an analysis of the elements and technique required for their production, would be very lengthy. Independent developments in allied fields which have been appropriated as part of the essential technique of experimental medicine, in themselves present, when enumerated, an imposing testimony of the comparative infinitesimal addition of the discoverer.

The apparatus and instruments with which the experimenter in medicine deals have become increasingly more precise and specialised due to advances in physics and mathematics and progress in medicine is contingent upon this fact. The experimenter today is entirely dependent upon and limited by the apparatus at his disposal: the microscope and all its accessories involving magnification, definition, illumination, and polarization, the ultra or dark field microscope, the slit ultra microscope, microtomes and their accessories, microchemical and other analytical balances, exact weights, thermometers and barometers, calorimeters, condensers, desiccators, stills, filters, sterilizers, pumps, blowers, burners, burettes, incubators, ammeters, galvanometers, rheostats, thermostats, viscosimeters, pipettes, micro-manipulator and many other indispensable instruments. His dependence upon mathematics is also revealed in his appropriation of the mathematical theory of probability and the mathematics of vital statistics.

Progress in experimental medicine is also directly correlated with advances in chemistry, bio-chemistry and bio-physics. The experimenter is dependent on chemistry for his reagents, for synthetic compounds, aniline dyes and vital stains, for his preservatives, and for the principle of specificity at the basis of the chemistry of immunity and serology. Bio-physics and bio-chemistry contribute to the fundamental equipment of the experimenter: the potentiometer and buffer solutions for measuring hydrogen-ion concentration, the measure of vitality and metabolism, the technique for the measurement of iso-electric point, osmotic pressure, and the accumulating data of colloid chemistry in all its phases. Knowledge in these interrelated fields has become so vast that many specialties have arisen, each requiring the investigation of experts. To pursue these investigations, they must draw upon, and are limited by, the existing knowledge already acquired by previous workers. When measured by the fund of accumulated knowledge from which they derive their data, any contribution they are likely to make, is minute.

An analysis of any phase of medicine at any period of its history will reveal a like dependence upon and limitation by, the existing knowledge in other fields.

CHAPTER III

Multiple Discoveries and Inventions in the History of Medicine

It is difficult to predict just when an invention or discovery in medicine will occur because all the necessary factors may exist in the cultural environment without the requisite new synthesis being made. Nevertheless, that invention is inevitable in medicine when the essential elements exist in culture, seems to be substantiated by the data derived from the many multiple inventions in the history of medicine, a list of which is appended. By inevitable is meant that the invention or discovery is not dependent upon the work of any one man but would have been made, and in these instances was made, independently by others. The invention or discovery must of course be made by human agency but not by any specific agent. The history of medicine could be written without the mention of names of persons now being extolled as being "responsible" for medical development.[1]

Bitter wrangles over priority of discovery and invention in medicine are familiar to even the most casual reader in the history of medicine.[2] The priority of a day, week or

---

[1] It may be urged that social praise is a necessary stimulus to provoke the assiduous and specialized research requisite for discovery in the field of medicine. But it is doubtful whether in the large majority of instances it is primarily expectation of fame and recognition which motivates men to engage in the studies which result in their discoveries.

[2] These have become so frequent that Dr. A. L. Soresi chairman of the historical section of the New York Academy of Medicine delivered a paper entitled "On the desirability of Instituting a Special Medical Board which should correspond to the Patent Office: The function of this medical board being to establish and protect the priority of ideas relating to medical subjects."

month is frequently decisive in determining who shall be called the inventor or discoverer, and credited with the honor attendant thereto. The claimants for priority accuse each other of confiscation and plagiarism of ideas, ignoring the manifest fact that all working from the same cultural base, from the same stock of knowledge, will reach similar conclusions upon independent inquiry. This discussion is not concerned with establishing claims of priority. Its purpose is to show that at approximately the same time men make the same discoveries and inventions in medicine independently of one another, because the existing culture contains the elements necessary for the invention.

A list of discoveries that have been made only once could be drawn up, but such a record would be of little significance. One could not conclude that these discoveries are of special importance, that they could not have been made a second time. When a discovery occurs and becomes widely known, all later studies which arrive at the same conclusions are considered merely corroborations of the original results. The rapidity with which such verifications follow the discovery is additional evidence of the fact that discoveries are only variations of prior knowledge, which would soon have been arrived at by other investigators in the same field. The discovery once made, in turn becomes part of the foundation upon which further researches are based.

Multiple inventions and discoveries are often accounted for by the phrase " necessity is the mother of invention ". This popular concept implies that a particular emergency provokes many men to concentrate on the same problem with the result that the discovery is made independently at approximately the same time more than once. In the history of medicine, little importance can be ascribed to necessity as a cause for a particular discovery because necessity is a constant not a variable factor. The necessity for effective cures was as urgent and potent among the primitive men as it is today; the best that they could do to combat disease was to use herbs and ascribe magic powers to the shaman. Man was helpless before the necessity of counteracting the plagues that ravaged Europe in the seventeenth century; necessity today does not enable him to cure cancer and other diseases of which he has no accurate knowledge and with which he is therefore unable to cope. Necessity, acting as a stimulus to research, cannot produce an invention or discovery without the existence of the essential elements in knowledge. It might therefore be said that in the history of medicine the variable factor, and therefore the cause of invention and discovery, is the existing knowledge or cultural base. The multiple discovery is not due to the sudden emergence of necessity but to the fact that the required elements previously absent or unappreciated are found in culture making the discovery possible.

Development in the fields of medicine and surgery is so gradual that it is difficult to determine just when to consider a discovery or invention as completed. It will be found that in the appended list of multiple inventions, some investigators described their findings with greater accuracy and thoroughness than others. The procedure has been to disregard this fact provided the independent discovery was essentially the same. When doubt entered as to the comparability of findings, the discovery or invention was not listed. The appended list is by no means complete, but is thought sufficient to prove the frequency of multiple invention and discoveries in the history of medicine.[1]

[1] The list of multiple inventions was compiled from the following books: F. H. Garrison, *History of Medicine*; J. H. Baas, *History of Medicine*; H. Drinkwater, *Fifty Years of Medical Progress*; D. Power and C. Thompson, *Chronologia Medica*; Frank Baker, "History of Anatomy" in *Reference Handbook of the Medical Sciences*, vol. i; Index Catalog, Surgeon General's Office, 1st, 2nd and 3rd Series; S. Gross, *History of*

A List of Some Multiple Discoveries and Inventions in the History of Medicine

I

Bulbo-urethral glands
    1684. Mery, Paris
    1699. Cowper, London

Duct of the parotid gland
    1655. Walter Needham, London
    1658. Nils Stensen, Copenhagen

Intestinal lymphatics and their connection with the thoracic duct
    1652. Jan Van Horne, Leyden
    1651. Olaus Rudbeck, Upsala
    1652. Joyliffe, England
    1653. Bartholinus, Denmark

Choriocapillary layer of the chorioid
    1702. Jacob Hovius, Treves on Rhine
           Ruysch, Amsterdam

Pupillary membrane
    1734. Albinus, Leyden
    1740. Von Wachendorff

Surgery; H. Billings, "History of Surgery" in Dennis, *System of Surgery*; W. Keen, *Sketch in the Early History of Anatomy and Surgery*; F. H. Garrison, "History of Pediatrics" in Abt's *Pediatrics*, vol. 1; Wright, *History of Laryngology and Rhinology*; *American Encyclopedia of Opthalmology*, vol. ix; Park, Williams and Krumwiede, *Pathogenic Microorganisms*; J. MacFarland, *Pathogenic Bacteria and Protozoa*; Muir and Ritchie, *Manual of Bacteria*; A. R. Guerard, "Bacteria" in *Reference Handbook of Medical Science*, vol. i; H. Vaquez, *Diseases of the Heart*; A. D. Hirshfelder, *Diseases of the Heart and Aorta*; G. D. Gibson, *Diseases of the Heart and Aorta*; L. T. Lord, *Diseases of the Bronchi, Lungs and Pleura*; W. N. Berkely, *Principles and Practice of Endocrine Medicine*; M. A. Starr, *Nervous Diseases, Organic and Functional*; W. Ogburn and D. Thomas "Are Inventions Inevitable," *Political Science Quarterly*, vol. xxxvii, no. 1; Periodical literature on specific diseases was also consulted.

Separable posterior elastic layer of the cornea
    1729. Benedict Duddell, London
    1769. Jean Descemet, Paris
    1769. Pierre Demours, Paris

Separation of facial and auditory nerves
    1794. Johann Christoph Mayer, Berlin and Leipsig
    1778. Samuel Thomas Soemmering, Bavaria

Tympanic nerve
    1775. Johann Ehrenritter, Vienna
    1811. L. L. Jacobson, Copenhagen

Distinction between motor and sensory roots of the spinal nerves
    1779. George Prochaska, Prague
    1816. Charles Bell, Edinburgh

Ciliary muscle
    1835. William Clay Wallace, New York
    1846. Brucke, Berlin
    1847. Bowman, Cheshire, England

Circular fibers
    1856. H. Mueller, Leipzig
    1839. W. C. Wallace, New York

Nerve fibers which pass from the cervical portion of the spinal cord to the cardiac plexus by way of the ganglia of the great sympathetic
    1812–30. Legallois, France
    1863. Von Bezold, Leipzig

Nerve cells in brain and spinal cord
    1833. Ehrenberg, Berlin
    1836. Valentin, Berne
    1836. Purkinje, Breslau and Prague

Axone of nerve cells
        Wagner, Göttingen
    1865. Deiters, Bonn

MULTIPLE INVENTIONS AND DISCOVERIES 113

Olfactory cells
    1862. Eckhardt, Giessen
    1862. Ecker, Freiburg
    1862. Max Schultz, Bonn

Taste buds
    1867. Schwalbe, Strassburg
    1867. Loven, Christiania

Skull composed of modified vertebrae
    1805. Oken, Jena
    1790. Goethe, Wiemar

Form of liver cells
    1838. Purkinje, Prague
    1838. Henle, Germany
    1838. Dutrochet, Paris

II

Lithotomy
    1756. Bond, Pennsylvania
    1760. Jones, New York

Ovariotomy
    1809. McDowell, United States
    1820. Chrysmar, Germany
    1821. N. Smith, United States
    1827. Galenzonski

Lithotripsy
    1830. Depeyre, New York
    1830. Spencer, Virginia
    1831. Randolph, Pennsylvania

Special uterine sounds
    1843. Huguier, France
    1843. Kiwisch, Prague
    1843. Simpson, Edinburgh

Hemostatic forceps
    1878. Koeberle, Alsace
    1878. Pean, Paris

Myomectomy of fibroid tumors of the uterus
    1844. Atlee, Pennsylvania
    1853. Burnham, Massachusetts
    1853. Kimball, Massachusetts

Tying of the diseased artery above the tumor
    1786. John Hunter, England
    1791. Desault, France

Interdental splint
    1866. Gunning, New York
    1866. Bean, Georgia

Excision of part of lower jaw in case of tumor
    1810. Deadrick, Tennessee
    1821. Smythe, New Orleans

Amputation of hip joint
    1806. Brashear, Kentucky
    1824. Mott, New York

Cholecystotomy
    1867. Bobbs, Indianapolis
    1878. Simms, Alabama

Gastro-enterostomy
    1881. Woelfler, Bohemia
    1881. Czerny, Freiburg

Ligating the appendix
    1885. W. Grant, Denver
    1885. Kroenlin, Switzerland

Removal of prostate by supra-pubic route
    1886. McGill, Leeds
    1888. Belfield, Chicago
    1896. Freyer, India

III

Description of adolescent apophysitis of the tibia
    1903. Osgood, Boston
    1903. Schlatter, Tübingen

Pseudo-coxalgia or Coxa Plana
    1910. Legg, United States
    1913. Perthes, Germany
    1913. Calve, France

Poliomyelitis transmitted to monkeys
    1909. Landsteiner and Popper, Germany
    1909. Flexner and Lewis, United States

Palsy from spinal deformity (caries)
    1779. Pott, London
    1779. David, France

IV

Laryngoscope
    1825. Latour, France
    1827. Senn, Geneva
    1829. Babington, London
    1832. Selliques, Paris
    1828. Baumes, Lyon
    1840. Liston, London
    1844. Avery, London
    1846. Eyrel, Vienna
    1854. Jacobi, New York
    1854. Garcia, London

Laryngeal paralysis
    1859. Turck, Vienna
    1860. Lewin, Germany
    1861. Mandl, France

Jackson-Avellis complex or syndrome
    1864. Jackson, London
    1891. Avellis, Berlin

Rosenbach-Semon law
    1880. Semon, London
    1880. Rosenbach, Breslau

Ogston-Luc operation
    1884. Ogston, England
    1896. Luc, France

Caldwell-Luc operation
    1893. Caldwell, United States
    1894. Spicer, England
    1897. Luc, France

Operation for deviated septum leaving the mucosa on both sides of the septum
    1899. Killian, Germany
    1903. Hagek, Germany
    1903. Menzel, Germany

V

Artificial Mydriasis
    1796. Leder, Jena
    1797. Reinarus, Hamburg
    1801. Himly, Bremen

Color blindness (Young-Helmholtz Theory)
    1807. Young, England
    1867. Helmholtz, Germany

Strabismus operation
    1818. Gibson, United States
    1839. Deffenbach, Berlin

Enlargement of the lachrymo-nasal canal at a single setting and throughout its whole extent
    1870. Williams, Cincinnati
    1870. Noyes, New York
    1876. Theobald, Baltimore

Opthalmoscope
    1847. C. Baggage, England
    1850. Helmholtz, Germany

Nature of the cataract
    1706. Brisseau, Donay
    1707. Maitre-Jan, Paris

VI

Plants composed of vesicles and rigid walls
    1665. Hooke, England
    1671. Grew, England
    1671. Malpighi, Bologna

Cellular basis of animal and plant tissue
    1824. Dutrochet, Paris
    1836. Valentin, Berne
    1837. Henle, Germany
    1838. Schwann, Germany
    1839. Turpin, Paris
    1839. Dumortier, Belgium
    1839. Purkinje, Prague
    1839. Müller, Berlin

Cell clump of nucleated protoplasm
    1835. Dujardin, France
    1838. Schleiden, Jena

Discovery of centrosome in the ovum
    1875. Flemming, Prague
    1876. Van Beneden, Brussels

VII

Theory of infection of microörganisms
    1546. Fracastoro, Verona
    1658. Kircher, Fulda
    1762. Plenciz, Vienna

Relation of microörganisms to fermentation and putrefaction
    1837. Schwann, Germany
    1837. Latour, France

Agglutination of typhoid fever
    1896. Gruenbaum, England
    1896. Widal, France

Separation of typhus from typhoid fever
    1837. Gerhard, Philadelphia
    1847. W. Jenner, London

Isolation of trichophyton tonsurans (ringworm)
    1842. Gruby, France
    1860. Hebra, Germany

Puerperal fever as a contagious disease
    1843. Holmes, United States
    1847. Semmelweiss, Vienna
    1858. Tarnier, Paris
    1875. Lister, England

Method of establishing pathogenic character of a given organism (Koch's Postulates)
    1840. Henle, Germany
    1877. Klebs, Koenigsberg
           Mitchell, United States

Pathology of traumatic infections
    1871. Klebs, Koenigsberg
    1878. Koch, Göttingen

Anthrax, causal relation
    1849. Pollender, Germany
    1850. Davaine, France

Anthrax, culture
    1871. Klebs, Koenigsberg
    1876. Koch, Germany
    1877. Pasteur, France

Immunity from anthrax by inoculation of virus
    1876. Toussaint, Toulouse
    1878. Pasteur, France
    1878. Sanderson and Greenfield, England

Typhoid fever as a contagious disease
    1865. Homan and Hartig, Norway
    1873. Budd, England

Amebic dysentery
    1860. Lambl, Prague
    1875. Lewis, Louisville, United States
    1875. Loesch, St. Petersburg
    1883. Koch and Gaffky, Egypt

Fourth Disease
  1886. Filatoff, Russia
  1900. Dukes, London
Discovery of parasite "actinomyces bovis" in man
  1845. Van Langenbeck, Germany
  1857–61. H. Lebert, France
  1868. Rivolta, Turin
  1871. Robin, France
  1875. Perroncito, Italy
  1878. J. Israel, Germany
Prevention of putrefaction of wounds by keeping germs from surface of wound
  1867. Lister, England
  1871. Guerini, United States
Constant occurrence of microörganisms in pyemic processes resulting from wound infection
  1866. Rindfleisch, Germany
  1871. Waldeyer, Germany
  1871. von Recklinghausen, Germany
  1880. Pasteur, France
  1881. Ogston, England
Mosquito as transmitter of yellow fever
  1848. J. C. Mott, South Carolina
  1853. Louis Daniel, Beauperthny
  1881. C. J. Finlay, Cuba
Causal relation of typhoid bacillus
  1880. Klebs, Koenigsberg
  1880. Eberth, Leipzig
  1880. Koch, Göttingen
Diphtheria bacillus
  1883. Klebs, Koenigsberg
  1884. Loeffler, Wurzburg
Meningococcus (Diplococcus intracellularis meningitidis)
  1884. Marchiafava and Celli, Italy
  1885. Leichtenstern, Germany
  1887. Weichselbaum, Germany

Glanders (bacillus mallei)
    1882. Bouchard, Capitan and Charin, France
    1882. Loeffler and Schütz, Germany
Bacilli in conjunctivitis (Koch-Weeks bacillus)
    1883. Koch, Germany
    1886. J. Weeks, United States
Bacillus coli (Escherich)
    1885. Emmerich, Germany
    1886. Escherich, Germany
Isolation of diplococcus of pneumonia
    1880. Sternberg, United States
    1880–1. Pasteur, France
Bubonic plague bacillus
    1894. Yersin, China
    1894. Kitasato, China
Spirochaeta vincenti
    1894. Plaut, Germany
    1896. Vincent, France
Morax-Axenfeld bacillus
    1896. Morax, France
    1896. Axenfeld, Germany
Influenza bacillus
    1892. Pfeiffer, Germany
    1892. Kitasato, Japan
    1892. Canon, Germany
Theory of filterable viruses
    1898. Loeffler and Frosch, Germany
    1899. Benjerink
Blastomyces dermatiti (Gilchrist and Stokes)
    1894. Busse, Germany
    1904. Gilchrist, United States
Isolation of bacillus aerogenes capsulatus
    1890. E. Fraenkel, Germany
    1892. Welch and Nuttal, United States
    1895. Kline, Germany
    1898. Beillon and Zuber, France

MULTIPLE INVENTIONS AND DISCOVERIES 121

Bacillus oedematiens
    1894. Novy, Germany
    1917. Weinberg and Seguin, France

Kala-Azar (Black sickness)
    1900. Leishman, Calcutta
    1903. Donovan, England
    1903. Wright, United States

Spirochete of relapsing fever
    1904. Ross and Milne, Uganda
    1904. Dutton and Todd, Congo State

Typhus fever produced in animals by inoculating with human blood
    1909. Nicolle, France
    1909. Anderson and Goldberger, United States

Bronchisepticus (Alkaligenes)
    1910. Ferry, United States
    1911. McGowan, United States

Spirochaeta Icterhemorrhagiae
    1915. Inado and Ido, Japan
    1915. Heubaner and Reiter, Germany
    1915. Uhlenhuth and Fromme, Germany

Transmissible lysis of bacteria (Bacteriophage)
    1915. Twort, England
    1917. d'Herelle, England

Vaccination
    1774. Jesty, England
    1781. Nash, England
    1781. Mrs. Randall. England
    1791. Jensen and Plett, Holstein
    1796. Jenner, England

Calf lymph obtained by inoculating the cow with human small pox
    1801. Gassner, Günsberg
    1839. Thiele, Russia
    1839. Ceeley, England
    1840. Badcock, England

Demonstration of pathological changes produced by the experimental injection of the toxins of diphtheria
    1891. Welch and Flexner, United States
    1891. Von Behring, Germany

Method of straining sputum for tubercle bacilli
    1882. Ziel, Germany
    1883. Nielsen, Germany

VIII

Aortic insufficiency
    1705. Cowper, England
    1695. Vieussens, Montpellier

Angina pectoris
    1768. Rougnon, France
    1768. Heberden, London

Heart-block (Stokes-Adams disease)
    1761. Morgagni, Venice
    1792. Spens, Edinburgh
    1827. Adams, Dublin
    1827. Burnett, England
    1846. Stokes, Dublin

Friction sound as sign of pericarditis
    1824. Collin, France
    1824. Devilliers, France

Insufficiency of the aortic value
    1829. Hodgkin, England
    1832. Corrigan, Dublin

Coexistence of cardiac hypertrophy with lesions of the kidney
    1827. Bright, England
    1839. Rayer, France
    1856. Traube, Germany

Orthostatic tachycardia
    1830. Graves, Dublin
    1838. Guy, London

MULTIPLE INVENTIONS AND DISCOVERIES

Pernicious anemia
    1849. Addison, London
    1869. Biermer, Zurich

Gallop rythm
    1847. Bouillard, France
    1858. Traube, Germany

Lead colic classed definitely among diseases attended by hypertension
    1895. Borgen, Germany
    1895. Potain, France

Effect of section of sympathethic was to paralyse and dilate the blood vessels
    1852. Brown-Sequard, America
    1852. Bernard, France
    1853. Waller and Budge, England

Sinus as the point of origin of normal excitations of the heart
    1900. Hering, Saxony
    1907. Rehfisch, Langendorff and Lehmann

Curves of the venous pulse (phlebograms)
    1867. Potain, France
    1894. Livierato, Italy

Classification of the arrhythmias
    1876. Riegel, Germany
    1880. See, France

Prolonged form of malignant endocarditis described
    1882. Jaccond, France
    1885. Osler, United States
    1901. Lenhartz, Germany

Sphygmomanometer with circular cuff
    1896. Riva-Rocci, Italy
    1897. Hill and Barnard, England

Paroxysmal tachycardia
    1889. Bouveret, France
    1889. Hoffman, Germany

Acquired pulmonary insufficiency
    1889. Dupre, France
    1890. Barie, France
    1892. Gerhardt, Germany

Necessary width of circular cuff of sphygmomanometer to secure constant results
    1906. von Recklinghausen, Germany
    1906. Weiss, France

IX

Stomach pump for the removal of opium and other poisons
    1822. Jukes, England
    1822. Bush, England

Pepsin as the active principle of gastric juice
    1835. Latour, France
    1833. Schwann, Louvain

X

Description of pulmonary blastomycosis
    1892. Wernicke, Buenos Aires
    1894. Busse, Germany
    1896. Gilchrist and Stokes, America

Hygienic dietetic treatment of phthisis
    1884. Dettweiler, Berlin
    1887. Brenner, Gorbersdorf

Disappearance of sputum of lobar pneumonia by absorption as a result of autolysis
    1901. F. Muller, Basel
    1901. Simon, Germany

Bottle aspirator for pleuritis
    1872. Potain and Castiaux, Paris
    1872. von Rasmussen, Copenhagen

Paravertbral triangle of dullness in pleuritis
    1897. Koranyi, Budapest
    1902. Grocco, Florence

Operation of paracentesis thoracis for pneumothorax
 1761. Monro, Scotland
 1766–67. Hewson, England

Solution of the problem of respiration
 1777. Priestly, Laeda
 1777. Scheele, Sweden
 1777. Spallanzani, Modena
 1777. Lavoisier, France

XI

Exophthalmic goitre (Graves' disease)
 1786–1825. Parry, Bath
 1800. Flajani, Italy
 1835. Graves, Dublin
 1840. von Basedow, Germany

Function of the pancreas
 1836. Purkinje, Prague
 1836. Pappenheim, Germany

Removal of enough of the pancreas in dogs to produce a glyscosuria "well marked persistent and accompanied by many other symptons of human diabetes"
 1889. Minkowski and Mering, Germany
 1889. de Dominicis, Italy

Chronic dyscrasia or insufficiency of the parathyroid glands as cause of eclampsia neonatorum
 1904. Lundborg, Stockholm
 1905. Berkeley, United States

Calcium salts arrest the spasms of parathyroid tetany
 1907. Parhon and Urechie, Roumania
 1908. Mac Callum and Voegtlin, United States

Adrenalin
 1897. Abel, United States
 1900. Takanine, United States
 1900. B. Moore, London
 1900. Furth, Strassburg
 1901. Aldrich, United States

XII

Correlation between dropsy and albuminous urine
    1811. Wells, London
    1813. Blackall, London

Benzoic acid changes to hippuric acid in urine
    1841. Ure, Edinburgh
    1842. Woehler, Germany

Beta oxybutyric acid in diabetic urine
    1884. Minkowski, Russia
    1884. Ed. Külz, Leipzig

XIII

Epilepsy (Jacksonian) described
    1836. Richard Bright, England
    1875. Jackson, England

Amaurotic family idiocy (Tay-Sachs disease)
    1880. Tay
    1887. Sachs, United States

Knee Jerk (Erb-Westphal's sign)
    1875. Erb, Bavaria
    1875. Westphal, Berlin

Disease of posterior columns of spinal cord
    1839. E. Stanley, London
    1856–58. Gull, England
    1858–59. Duchenne, Paris

" Intentional tremor " as differential sign of multiple sclerosis
    1860. B. Cohn, Berlin
    1886. Charcot, France

Asthenic bulbar paralysis or myasthenia gravis
    1685. Willis, England
    1878. Erb, Bavaria
    1893. Goldflam, Leipzig

Progressive muscular atrophy
    1886. Marie and Charcot, France
    1886. Tooth, England

XIV

Red corpuscles described
    1658. Swammerdam, Amsterdam
    1665. Malpighi, Bologna

Method of injecting blood vessels with wax
    1665. Ruysch, Hague
    1677. Swammerdam, Amsterdam

Bacterial effect of blood serum
    1888. Nuttall, San Francisco
    1889. Buchner, Jena

Transfusion of alien blood
    1654. Folli
    1665–67. Lower, London
    1667. Denys, Paris

XV

Chloroform
    1831. Soubeiran, Paris
    1831. Guthrie, New York
    1832. von Liebig, Darmstadt

Sulphuric ether as an anesthetic
    1842. Long, Georgia
    1846. Liston, London
    1846. Morton, Massachusetts
    1846. Jackson, Massachusetts
    1847. Pirogoff, Russia

Cocaine as an anesthetic
    1870–84. V. K. Anrep, Bonn
    1884. Koller, Germany

Sulphonal
    1884. Baumann, Strassburg
    1888. Kast, Berlin

Syringe for hypodermic injection
    1845. Rynd, Dublin
    1851. Pravas, France
    1855. Wood, Edinburgh

BIBLIOGRAPHY

Baker, Frank, History of Anatomy, *Reference Handbook of the Medical Sciences*, 3rd ed., New York, 1913, i, 323-345.
——, The Two Sylviuses, *Johns Hopkins Hospital Bulletin*, 1909, xx, 329-339.
Bailey, James Blake, *The Diary of a Resurrectionist*, London, 1896.
Bass, Johann, *History of Medicine*, translated by H. E. Henderson, New York, 1889.
Bayard, A., *Influence de la Vaccin sur la Population*, Paris, 1856.
Begbie, J. W., Early History of Anatomy, *Edinburgh Medical Journal*, 1868, xiv, part 1, 97-113.
Berkely, William N., *Principles and Practice of Endocrine Medicine*, New York, 1926.
Billings, John S., History and Literature of Surgery, Dennis, Frederic, *System of Surgery*, Philadelphia, 1895, I, 9-144.
Birch, John, *Letter Occasioned by the Many Failures of Cow Pox*, London, 1805.
——, *Serious Reasons for Uniformily Objecting to the Practice of Vaccination*, London, 1806.
British Ministry of Health, *Small Pox and Vaccination*, London, 1921.
British Royal Commission on Vaccination. Reports with Minutes of Evidence and Appendices, i-vi, London, 1889-1897; Final Report and Appendices, London, 1896-1897.
Brown, Thomas, *Inquiry into the Anti-Variolous Power of Vaccination*, Edinburgh, 1809.
Butler, George F., Cubism in Medicine, *Illinois Medical Journal*, 1921, xxxix, 250-256.
Camac, Charles N., *Epoch Making Contributions to Medicine, Surgery and Allied Sciences*, Philadelphia, 1909.
Cameron, Charles A., *History of the Royal College of Surgeons in Ireland*, Dublin, 1886.
Cannon, Walter B., *Anti-vivisection Legislation: Its History, Aims and Menace*, Chicago, 1913.
——, *Some Characteristics of Anti-vivisection Literature*, Chicago, 1911.
Chaplin, Arnold, Medicine in the Century Before Harvey, *British Medical Journal*, 1922, ii, 707-712.
Cheyne, Watson, *Lister and His Achievement*, London, 1925.

Civilization in the United States, edited by Harold E. Stearns, New York, 1912.
Comrie, John D., Early Anatomical Instruction at Edinburgh, *Edinburgh Medical Journal*, 1922, xxix, 273-296.
Copeland, Edgar P., Leopold Auenbrugger, *Virginia Medical Semi-Monthly*, Richmond, 1914, xix, 94-98.
Cordell, Eugene F., Charles Frederick Wiesenthal, *Johns Hopkins Hospital Bulletin*, 1900, xi, 170-174.
Cow Pox Chronicle, London, 1808-1810.
Crawfurd, Raymond, Forerunners of Harvey in Antiquity, *British Medical Journal*, 1919, ii, 551-556.
Creswell, C. H., Anatomy in the Early Days, *Edinburgh Medical Journal*, 1919, n. s., xii, 141-156.
Daglish, John, *Practical Observations on Vaccine Innoculation*, Newcastle, 1825.
De Back, James, *Discourse of, in which he handles the nullity of spirits, Sanguification, the heat of living things*, London, 1673.
De Kruif, Paul, *Microbe Hunters*, New York, 1926.
———, *Our Medicine Men*, New York, 1922.
Descour, L., *Pasteur and His Work*, translated by A. F. and B. H. Wedd, London, 1922.
Donley, J. Riolan and Harvey, *Annals of Medical History*, New York, 1923, v, 26-33.
Dowie, J. A., Doctors, *Drugs and Devils or the Foes of Christ the Healer*, Zion City., Ill., 1901.
Drinkwater, Harry, *Fifty Years of Medical Progress, 1873-1922*, London, 1924.
Duckworth, Dyce, Rational Empiricism and Scientific Medicine, *British Medical Journal*, 1911, i, 1217-1221.
Dukes, Cuthbert, *Lord Lister*, London, 1924.
Encyclopedia Brittanica, 11th ed., 1911, xvi, 777-9; xxiv, 631.
Fischer, George, *Chirurgie vor 100 Jahren*, Leipsig, 1876.
Fleming, George, *Pasteur and His Work*, London, 1886.
Flexner, A., *Medical Education in Europe*, New York, 1912.
———, *Medical Education in the United States and Canada*, New York, 1910.
Frank, Mortimer, Medical Instruction in the Seventeenth Century, *Journal of American Medical Association*, 1915, lxiv, 1373-1380.
Garrison, Fielding H., *History of Medicine*, Philadelphia, 2nd ed., 1917, 3rd ed., 1921.
———, History of Pediatrics, Abt's *Pediatrics*, Philadelphia. 1923, i, 1-170.
———, In Defence of Vesalius, *Bulletin Society Medical History Chicago*, 1916, i, no. 4, 47-65.

Gibbs, John, *Compulsory Vaccination*, London, 1856.
Gibson, George A., *Diseases of the Heart and Aorta*, Edinburgh, 1898.
Giddings, Franklin H., *Studies in the Theory of Human Society*, New York, 1922.
Godlee, Rickman J., *Lord Lister*, London, 1917.
Goldson, William, *Cases of Small Pox Subsequent to Vaccination*, Portsea, 1804.
Gould, George M., Reception of Medical Discoveries, *Annals of American Opthalmology*, 1904, xiii.
Grissom, Eugene, *Medical Science in Conflict with Materialism*, Wilmington, N. C., 1880.
Gross, Samuel D., History of Surgery, *A Century of American Medicine, 1776-1876*, Philadelphia, 1876.
———, *Lives of Eminent American Physicians and Surgeons of the Nineteenth Century*, Philadelphia, 1861.
Guerard, Arthur R., Bacteria, *Reference Handbook of the Medical Sciences*, New York, 3rd ser., 1913, i, 825-876.
Gunn, Robert A., *Vaccination, Its Fallacies and Evils*, New York, 1882.
Harris, David F., Harvey versus Caespinus, *17th International Congress of Medicine, Proceedings of the Section on the History of Medicine*, London, 1913, xxiii, 351-356.
———, History of the Events which Led to the Passing of the Anatomy Act, *Canadian Medical Journal*, 1920, x, 283-4.
Hartwell, Edward M., Hindrances to Anatomical Studies in United States, *Annals of Anatomy and Surgery*, 1881, iii, 209-225.
———, Study of Human Anatomy, Historically and Legally Considered, *Johns Hopkins University, Studies from the Biological Laboratory*, 1883, ii, 65-116.
Harvey, William, *An Anatomical Disquisition on the Motion of the Heart and Blood*, Willis Translation, London, 1847.
———, *Second Disquisition to John Riolan*, London, 1847.
Hirschfelder, Arthur D., *Diseases of the Heart and Aorta*, Philadelphia, 3rd ed., 1918.
Holmes, Samuel J., *Louis Pasteur*, New York, 1924.
Index Catalog, Surgeon General's Office, Washington.
Jacobi, Abraham, *Rudolph Virchow*, New York, 1881.
Jacobson, Arthur C., Robert Knox and the Resurrectionists, *Interstate Medical Journal*, St. Louis, 1915, xxii, 462-472.
Journal American Medical Association, editorials, 1921, lxxvii, 792-3, 1922, lxxix, 1448-9.
Keen, William W., *A Sketch of the Early History of Practical Anatomy*, Philadelphia, 1874.
———, *The Influence of Anti-vivisection on Character*, Chicago, 1912.

BIBLIOGRAPHY

Kelly, Howard A. and Burrage, Walter L., *American Medical Biographies*, Baltimore, 1920.
Klebs, Arnold C., Leonardo da Vinci and his Anatomical Studies, *Bulletin of the Society of Medical History Chicago*, 1916, i, no. 4, 66-83.
Lancet, London, 1875, ii, 597.
——, 1877, i, 361.
Leverson, Montague R., *Pasteur the Plagiarist*, London, 1911.
Lipscomb, George, *A Dissertation on the Failure and Mischiefs of the Disease Called the Cow Pox*, London, 1805.
——, *Cow Pox Exploded, or the Inconsistencies, Absurdities and Falsehoods of Some of its Defenders Exposed*, London, 1806.
——, *Innoculation for the Small Pox Vindicated*, London, 1805.
Lister, Joseph B., *Collected Works*, Oxford, 1908-9.
London Society for the Abolition of Compulsory Vaccination, Annual Report, 1886.
Longcope, Warfield, Milestones in Medicine, *Educational Review*, 1916, lii, 338-48.
Lord, Frederick T., *Diseases of the Bronchi, Lungs and Pleura*, 2nd ed., Philadelphia, 1925.
Lovett, William, *Life and Struggles*, vol. i, Knopf ed., New York, 1920.
MacFarland, J., *Pathogenic Bacteria and Protozoa*, 9th ed., Philadelphia and London, 1919.
McMurrich, J. P., Leonardo da Vinci and Vesalius, *Medical Library and Historical Journal*, Brooklyn, 1906, iv, 338-350.
Medical and Physical Journal, London, 1799-1814.
Medical Observer, London, 1807-1810.
Meigs, Charles D., *Memoir of S. G. Morton*, Philadelphia, 1851.
Merry, Joseph, *A Conscious View of the Circumstances and Proceedings Respecting Vaccine Innoculation*, Bath, 1800.
Metchnikoff, Olga, *Life of Elie Metchnikoff*, Boston and New York, 1921.
Mitchell, S. Weir, The Early History of Instrumental Precision in Medicine, *Transactions of Congress of American Physicians*, New Haven, 1891, ii, 159-181.
Moon, Robert H., *The Relation of Medicine to Philosophy*, London, 1909.
Moseley, Benjamin, *An Oliver for a Roland*, London, 1807.
——, *Medical Tracts*, London, 1799.
——, *Review of the Report of the Royal College of Physicians on Vaccination*, 2nd ed., London, 1808.
——, *Treatise on Lues Bovilla*, London, 1805.
Muir, Robert and Ritchie, James, *Manual of Bacteriology*, 6th ed., New York, 1913.
Neuburger, Max, *Leopold Auenbrugger*, Vienna, 1922.
New York Anti-vaccination Society, *Tracts*, 1926.

BIBLIOGRAPHY

Ogburn, William F., *Social Change*, New York, 1923.
Ogburn, William and Thomas, Dorothy, Are Inventions Inevitable? A Note on Social Evolution, *Political Science Quarterly*, 1922, xxxvii, 83-99.
Otis, Edward O., Auenbrugger and Laennec, *Boston Medical and Surgical Journal*, 1898, cxxxix, 281-285.
Packard, Francis R., Early British Resurrectionists, *Medical News*, New York, 1902, lxxxi, 67-73.
——, *History of Medicine in the United States*, Philadelphia, 1901.
Park, William H., Williams, Anna W. and Krumwiede, Charles, *Pathogenic Microörganisms*, 8th ed., Philadelphia, 1924.
Payne, J. F., Thomas Addison, *Dictionary of National Biography*, New York and London, 1908, i, 133-4.
Power, D'Arcy, A Revised Chapter in the Life of Dr. William Harvey, *Proceedings of Royal Society of Medicine, Section on the History of Medicine*, 1916-17, x, 33-70.
——, *William Harvey*, New York, 1898.
Power, D'Arcy and Thompson, C. J. S., *Chronologia Medica*, New York, 1923.
Puschman, Theodor, *History of Medical Education*, translated and edited by Evan H. Hare, London, 1891.
Ring, John, *A Roland for an Oliver*, London, 1807.
Robinson, Victor, *Pathfinders in Medicine*, New York, 1912.
Rogers, W. R., *Examination of Cow Pox Evidence*, London, 1805.
Rolleston, Humprey, The Reception of Harvey's Doctrine of the Circulation of the Blood in England as Exhibited in the Writings of Two Contemporaries, *Essays on the History of Medicine Presented to Karl Sudhoff*, 1924.
Roth, M., *Andreas Vesalius Bruxellensis*, Berlin, 1892.
Rowley, William, *Cow Pox Innoculation No Security Against Small Pox Infection, With Above Five Hundred Proofs of Failure. To which are added the modes of treating the beastly new diseases produced from cow pox. Explained by two coloured copper plate engravings and five hundred dreadful cases of small pox after vaccination or Cow Pox Mange, Cow Pox Ulcers, Cow Pox Evils or Abscess, Cow Pox Mortification. With the author's certain experienced and successful mode of Innoculating for small pox which now becomes necessary from cow pox failure*, 3rd ed., London, 1806.
Shastid, Thomas H., History of Opthalmology, *American Encyclopedia of Opthalmology*, Chicago, 1917, xi, 8524-8904.
Shaw, George Bernard, *Back To Methuselah*, Preface, New York, 1921.
——, *The Doctor's Dilemma*, Preface, New York, 1906.
Shillito, Charles, *Cases of Cow Pox Failures and Mischiefs*, London, 1808.

Sinclair, William J., *Semmelweis, His Life and Doctrine*, Manchester, 1909.
Simpson, L. Y., *Landmarks in the Struggle Between Science and Religion*, London, 1925.
Singer, Charles, A Medical Compendium of the First Half of the Twelfth Century, *Bulletin Society Medical History Chicago*, 1917, ii, 53-96.
——, *Evolution of Anatomy*, London, 1925.
Smith, Stephen, Reminiscences of Two Epochs—Anaesthesia and Asepsis, *Johns Hopkins Hospital Bulletin*, 1919, xxx, 273-278.
Spencer, Herbert, *Social Statics*, New York.
Spielman, H. M., *Iconography of Andreas Vesalius*, London, 1925.
Squirell, R., *Observations Addressed to the Public in General on the Cow Pox, shewing that it originates in scrophula, commonly called the evil. Illustrated with cases to prove that it is no security against the small pox. Also pointing out the dreadful consequences of the new disease so recently introduced into the human constitution. To which are added, observations on the small pox innoculation, proving it to be more beneficial to society than the vaccine*, London, 1805.
Starr, Moses A., *Nervous Diseases, Organic and Functional*, 4th ed., New York, 1913.
Steiner, O. S., Surgical Fads and Fancies, *Ohio State Medical Journal*, 1921, xvii, 170-2.
Stern, Bernhard J., *Should We Be Vaccinated: A Survey of the Controversy in its Historical and Scientific Aspects*, New York, 1927.
Streeter, Edward C., The Role of Certain Florentines in the History of Anatomy, Artistic and Practical, *Johns Hopkins Hospital Bulletin*, 1916, xxvi, 113-118.
Struthers, John, *Historical Sketch of the Edinburgh Anatomical School*, Edinburgh, 1867.
Tondorf, F., *The Vindication of Vivisection*, Washington, 1920.
Vaccination Inquirer, London.
Vallery-Radot, Rene, *Life of Pasteur*, translated by Mrs. R. I. Devonshire, New York, 1924.
Vaquez, Henri, *Diseases of the Heart*, translated and edited by George F. Laidlow, Philadelphia, 1924.
Verdi-Delisle, *De la degenerescence physique et morale de l'espece humaine determinee par le Vaccin*, Paris, 1855.
Wallace, Alfred Russel, *Vaccination a Delusion, Its Penal Enforcement a Crime*, London, 1898.
Walsh, J. J., *History of Medicine in New York*, New York, 1919.
——, *The Popes and Science*, New York, 1908.
Weir, Robert F., *On the Antiseptic Treatment of Wounds*, New York, 1878.

White, Andrew, *The Warfare of Science*, New York, 1876.
Wilkinson, J. J. Garth, *Pasteur and Jenner, An Example and a Warning*, London, 1883.
Willis, Robert, *Works of Harvey*, London, 1847.
Wood, Zachary, *Preface to Harvey's Anatomical Exercises*, London, 1673.
Wrench, Guy T., *Lord Lister*, London, 1914.
Wright, Jonathan, *History of Laryngology and Rhinology*, 2nd ed., Philadelphia, 1914.
Wynn, F. B., Fads and Fancies of Medical Practice, *Journal of Indiana State Medical Association*, 1921, xiv, 117-123.
Young, Sidney, *Annals of the Barber-Surgeons*, London, 1890.

INDEX

Anatomy, and dissection, 34 *et seq.*, 100-101; multiple discoveries in history of, 111-113
Anesthesia, 26
Anthrax, 74 *et seq.*, 104
Antisepsis, 8, 29, 80 *et seq.*, 93, 94
Anti-vaccinationists, 53 *et seq.*, 78 *et seq.*
Asepsis, 8, 29, 90 et seq., 93, 94
Auenbrugger, 25, 51 *et seq.*, 94
Authority, 13, 16, 18, 25, 33, 43-44, 50, 52, 62, 69, 79, 89, 93

Biography in medical history, 7, 8, 97 *et seq.*
Blood, multiple discoveries in study of, 127
Bloodletting, 24, 28
"Body snatching", 39 *et seq.*
"Burking", 42

Church, and dissection, 28, 35 *et seq.*; and evolution, 28
Circulation of the blood, 8, 44 *et seq.*
Cliques in medical profession, 30, 33, 72
Conflict between phases of culture, 17, 18, 19, 29, 50, 52, 65, 79, 89, 94
Conservatism in medicine, 8, 11, 20 *et seq.*
Cultural factors retarding diffusion, 18, 33, 43, 50, 52, 65, 70, 79, 89, 92, 94
Culture defined, 8

Dependence on existing knowledge, 7, 8, 100 *et seq.*
Dissection, 8, 32, 34 *et seq.*, 93; Company of Barber Surgeons and, 38; church and, 28, 35 *et seq.*; Galenic tradition and, 37; Greek, 34-35; history of, 100-101; legislation and, 38; of live bodies, 39, 40, 43; religious attitudes affecting, 34

Drugs, multiple discoveries in history of, 127
Drug therapy, status of, 21 *et seq.*

Education, 13
Endocrinology, multiple discoveries in history of, 125
Experimental method, opposition to, 43, 50, 52

Fads in medicine, 24, 32
Fear, 12, 17, 18, 19, 39, 50, 55, 61, 65, 89, 93
Fermentation, 73, 104
Folk medicine, 32

Galen, 28, 37 *et seq.*, 43, 44, 47, 49, 50
Germ theory, 74, 81 *et seq.*
Gynecology, fashions in, 23

Habit, 12, 14, 18, 27, 33, 43, 50, 52, 65, 70, 79, 88, 89, 93
Harvey, Wm., 25, 44 *et seq.*, 97, 102 *et seq.*
Heart, multiple discoveries in treatment of diseases of, 122-123
Hippocrates, 51, 52, 97
Holmes, O. W. 26, 66 *et seq.*

Identification, psychological principle of, 32, 34, 42, 77
Ignorance, 12, 18, 19, 31, 33, 39, 43, 50, 52, 60 *et seq.*, 65, 70, 79, 89, 93
Inevitability of invention and discovery, 108
Introduction, 7 *et seq.*

Jenner, Edward, 30, 53, 56-60, 65, 77-8, 103

Knowledge and receptiveness, 12

Laryngology, multiple discoveries in history of, 115-116

135

INDEX

Lister, Joseph, 26, 68, 74, 80 *et seq.*, 90, 105
Lungs, multiple discoveries in treatment of diseases of, 124

Masses, part played by, in medical conservatism, 31, 33, 79
Money, role of, 13, 17, 18, 29, 31, 88-9

Necessity and invention, 108-109
Nervous diseases, multiple discoveries in treatment of, 126

Ogburn, William F., 11; and D. Thomas, 111
Ophthalmology, multiple discoveries in history of, 116
Orthopedics, multiple discoveries in history of, 114-5

Mechanical factors retarding diffusion, 13, 16, 18, 33, 43, 50, 52, 65, 92, 94
Medicine, as a science, 20 *et seq.*, 33
Multiple inventions and discoveries in history of medicine, 8, 108 *et seq.*

Pain and unpleasant, avoidance of, 14, 16, 18, 19, 32, 42, 60, 62, 65, 80, 89, 93
Parasitology, multiple discoveries in history of, 117-122
Pasteur, 8, 30, 32, 71 *et seq.*, 76, 81, 94, 97, 98, 104, 105
Patent medicine manufacturers, propaganda of, 32, 33, 55, 62
Pediatrics, 23
Percussion, 8, 51 *et seq.*, 94

Personality conflicts retarding diffusion, 15, 17, 18, 30-1, 33, 58, 59, 65, 71, 89, 94
Power of tradition, 28, 69, 73
Priority, 15, 69, 70, 76, 89, 108-9
Psychological factors retarding diffusion, 18, 19, 33, 42, 50, 52, 64, 65, 70, 79, 89, 92, 93
Puerperal fever, 8, 26, 66 *et seq.*

Quacks, 24, 32, 55

Rationalization, 14, 18, 34, 42, 60, 61, 65, 93
Resurrectionists, 41 *et seq.*

Semmelweis, Ignatz, 26, 66 *et seq.*, 105
Social Pressure, 14 *et seq.*, 18, 43, 50, 59, 70, 76, 79, 88-89, 93
Stomach, multiple discoveries in treatment of diseases of, 124
Summary, 93 *et seq.*
Surgery, fashions in, 24; multiple discoveries in history of, 113-114
Survivals, 14

Vaccination, 8, 28, 31, 53 *et seq.*, 93, 94, 103 *et seq.*; individual liberty and, 63-65; religious opposition to, 63; Royal Commission on, 55, 62-64; sanitation and, 62 *et seq.*, 65
Vesalius, 36, 37 *et seq.*, 100 *et seq.*, 103
Vested interests, 12, 16, 33, 79; economic, 11, 12, 18, 19, 28, 29, 32, 33, 43, 55, 56, 62, 63, 65, 75, 89, 94; psychological, 18, 27, 33, 50, 52, 64, 79, 89, 90, 93
Vivisection, 32, 47, 50, 77 *et seq.*, 79

Bei Fragen zur Produktsicherheit wenden Sie sich bitte an:
If you have any questions regarding product safety,
please contact:

Walter de Gruyter GmbH
Genthiner Straße 13
10785 Berlin
productsafety@degruyterbrill.com